the successful face

By
AMY GREENE

Coauthor
MOLLY POMERANCE

Designed by
MIKI DENHOF

Illustrated by
L. WEISBERG

Foreword by
GERALDINE STUTZ

SUMMIT BOOKS NEW YORK

Published by SUMMIT BOOKS
A Division of Simon & Schuster, Inc.
Simon & Schuster Building
1230 Avenue of the Americas
New York, New York 10020
SUMMIT BOOKS and colophon are trademarks of Simon & Schuster, Inc.
Manufactured in the United States of America
1   3   5   7   9   10   8   6   4   2
Library of Congress Cataloging in Publication Data
Greene, Amy.
The successful face.
1. Beauty, Personal.   2. Face—Care and hygiene.
3. Cosmetics.   4. Hairdressing.   I. Title.
RA778.G8   1985   646.7'26   85-14672
ISBN: 0-671-54772-0

Photo credits
Kathryn Abbe, pp. 20–21
Joshua Greene, pp. 14, 16, 17, 60, 61, 96, 97
Jill Krementz © p. 12

For Joshua and Anthony,
with all my love;
and to Miki, Molly and Geraldine—
colleagues, comrades in arms,
friends.

ACKNOWLEDGMENTS

To start at the beginning, I must go back to my years at *Glamour* magazine, for whom I developed the "makeover." This could not have been done without the blessing of Condé Nast's S. I. Newhouse, Alexander Lieberman and Kathleen Casey, then editor in chief of *Glamour*. They gave me my career.

Beauty Checkers—Makeovers in Action—became a reality fifteen years ago at Henri Bendel in New York City. It could never have been born without the generous help of Sammy Davis Jr., my friend of thirty-two years and a gentleman to his toes. My other indispensable friend, adviser and pillar of strength was—and still is—Geraldine Stutz, president of Henri Bendel and the greatest merchant in retailing then, now and always.

I owe the continuing success of Beauty Checkers to the loyalty, skill, hard work and sensitivity of my staff.

With *The Successful Face,* the makeover has come full circle. We are once again in print, this time in hardcover (and available for a mini-series). For this project, I want to thank the extraordinary professionals at Summit Books—Wendy Nicholson, associate publisher, a well of ideas and enthusiasm; Jim Silberman, publisher, who was right; and Ileene Smith, my beloved editor, who initiated this book through her curiosity and whose feel for words is brilliant.

Thanks from my heart to L. Weisberg, our splendid artist who remained undaunted by all we asked her to do.

To Lisa Palmer, our "Before and After," whose sense of humor and graciousness are unparalleled.

To Dr. Mark Podwal, our skin guru, for his help.

To Ruth Pomerance, for endless hours of research in dingy, dusty movie still archives.

And to Molly Pomerance, for her invaluable patience, ability to turn on a dime, awesome knowledge of the English language, total commitment to this project and deep lasting friendship.

Finally, my gratitude to Miki Denhof, my art director and dearest friend, who has brought her unique artistic vision to *The Successful Face.* With her wealth of culture, skill and experience, she has worked tirelessly to bring this book to fruition.

Thank God they are all an integral part of my life.

CONTENTS

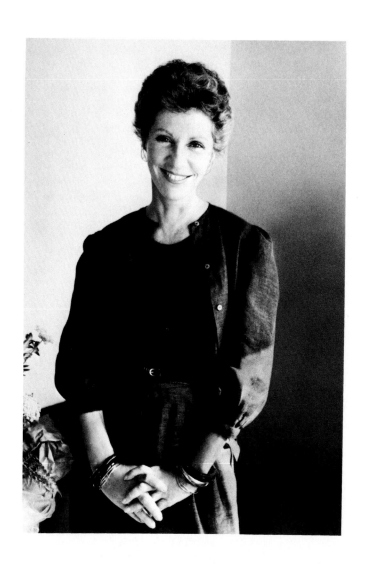

FOREWORD

amy Greene began making marvelous faces when she was the shining star beauty editor of *Glamour* magazine. She gave the makeover mass appeal—and filled her pages with before and after pictures that proved what near miracles the correct makeup, properly applied, could perform.

It was, of course, a brilliant breakthrough idea—one that earned for Amy a singular shimmering status in the beauty firmament. And eventually brought her to Bendel's—where it has been our long-running good luck to be Beauty Checkers' home base.

The Beauty Checkers concept is a natural extension of Amy's magazine makeovers. It offers show and tell makeup sessions that teach women to put their best faces forward. The approach is clear, concise and complete—as you'll find for yourself in the pages that follow. Because *The Successful Face* is really a foolproof beauty manual—and proof positive of the extraordinary no nonsense know how that has made Amy such a boon to us at Bendel's.

Geraldine Stutz
New York City, May 1985

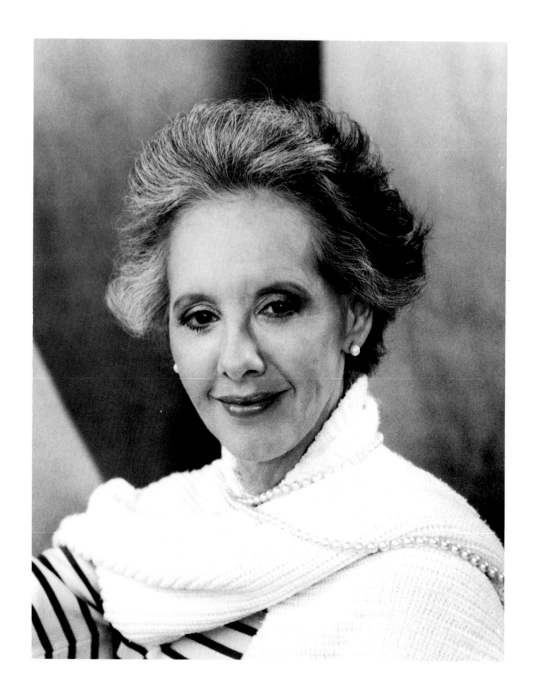

INTRODUCTION

ever since Eve, women have been fascinated by the way they look—and frustrated by their inability to reach their ideal. For the past fifteen years at Beauty Checkers at Henri Bendel in New York City, I have been showing women exactly how to do this, using the makeup they bring with them. *The Successful Face* is the logical extension of Beauty Checkers. At last—in response to thousands of requests—you can take me home with you.

Just follow the bouncing ball and you'll find everything falling into place. Makeovers are straightforward. Keep your efforts simple until they become routine. Making up is very much like cooking: There is no mystery; the basic ingredients are always the same.

The Successful Face offers clear, concise knowledge and advice without stress, complication or undue drama. Like a Beauty Checkers customer, when you have read this book you will know exactly how to look your best, every day of your life.

Amy Greene
New York City, May 1985

BEFORE

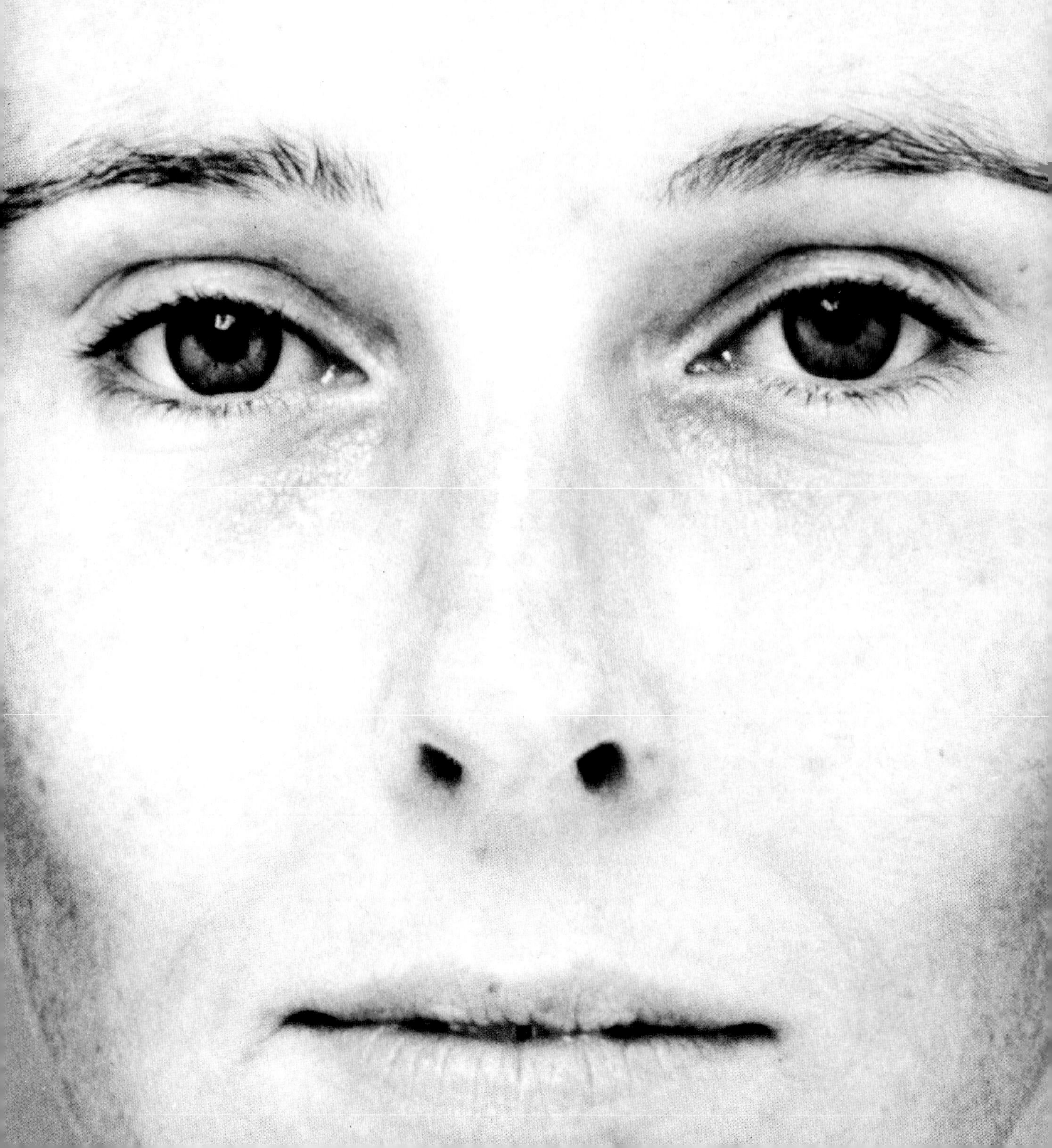

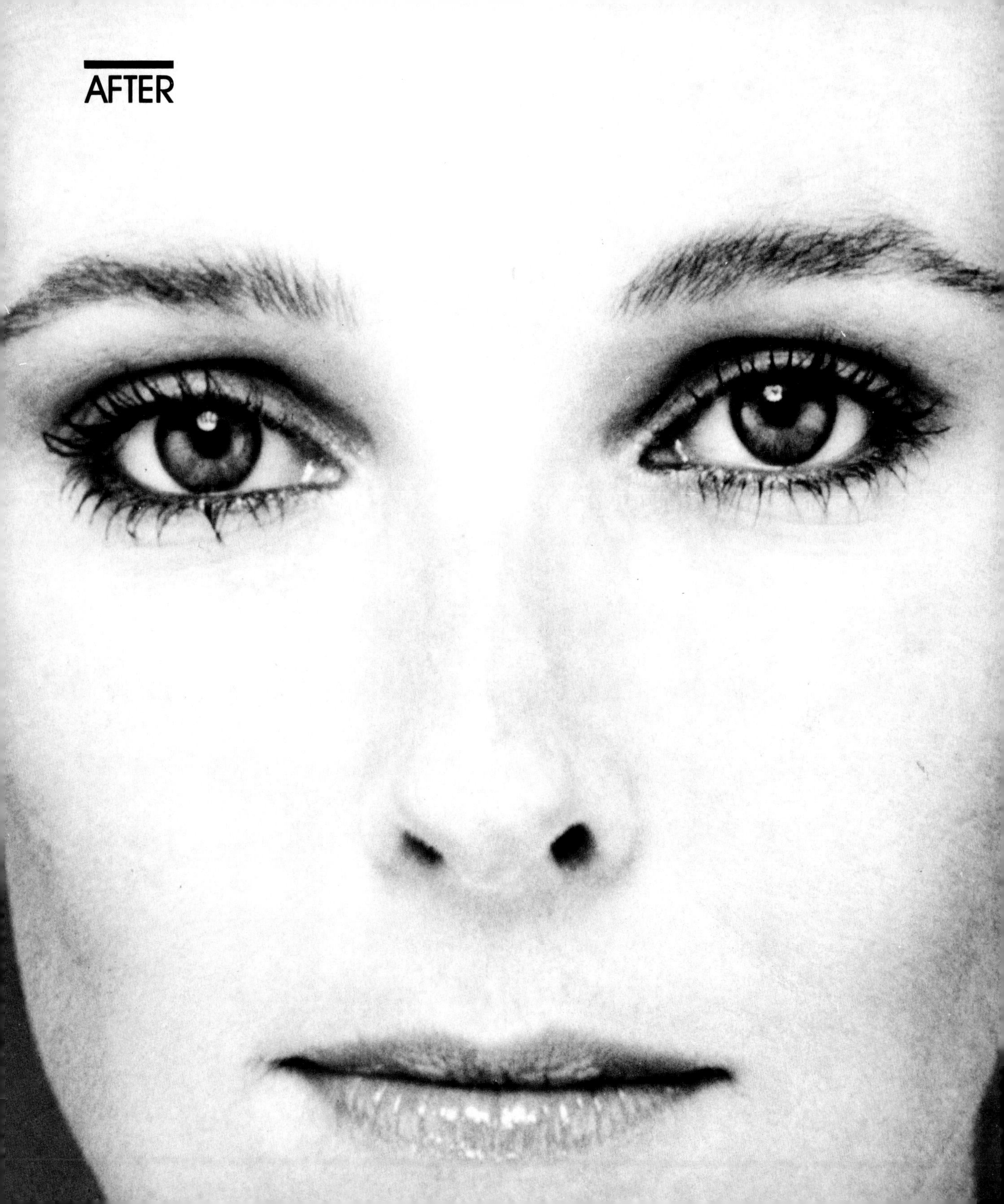
AFTER

your face

THE BEGINNING

You've got ten minutes. You're due at your first board meeting early this morning. You look in the mirror. What do you see? Certainly not Botticelli's Venus.

     "Come on, it's not that bad. Now, make each minute count."

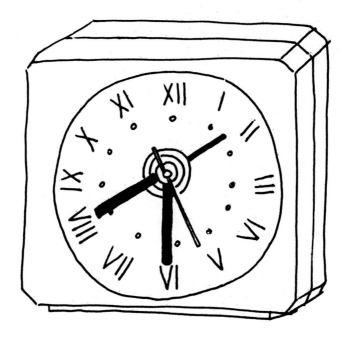

Everyone's face is entitled to ten minutes.

1. The first thing to do: Splash your face with lukewarm water.

2. Then moisturize. Did you know you should always apply moisturizer to a damp face?

3. Neutralize—to tone down sallowness or ruddiness, nature's imperfections. A tiny dot goes far.

4. Apply foundation—to refine skin texture.

5. Apply darkness concealer—anywhere you need it.

6. Put on mascara—the one essential eye makeup.

7. Powder face all over—to set everything for several hours.

8. Apply blusher—suck in cheeks, color on cheekbones. Instant pick me up.

9. Put on lipstick—and smile, probably the first of the day.

10. Bend forward. Brush hair —to bring it back to life.

Seems like a lot? But admit it: Don't you actually look better? And you even have a few minutes to spare!

For a full description of all your basic steps and techniques, turn to the following pages.

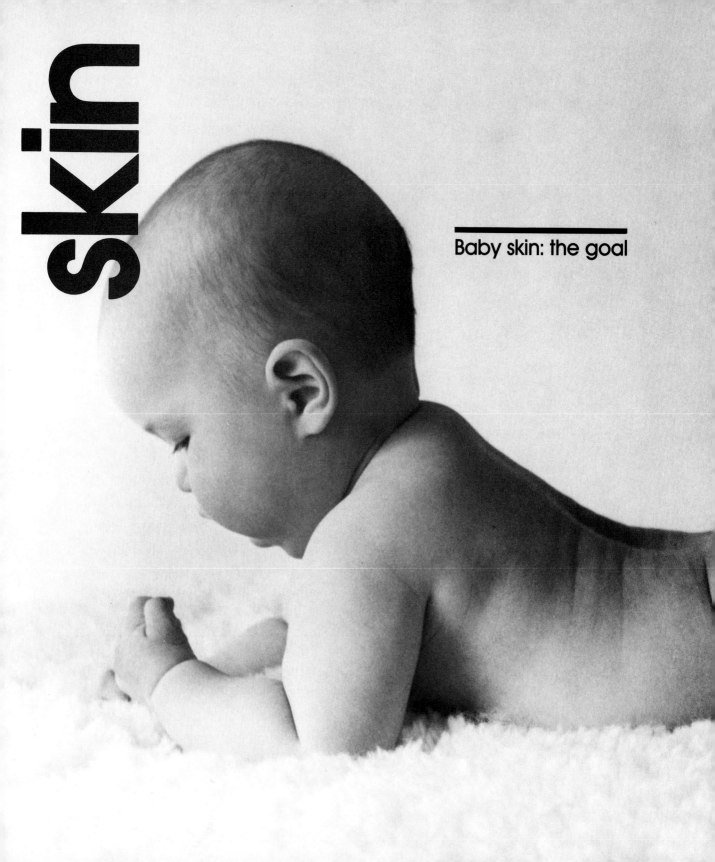

skin

Baby skin: the goal

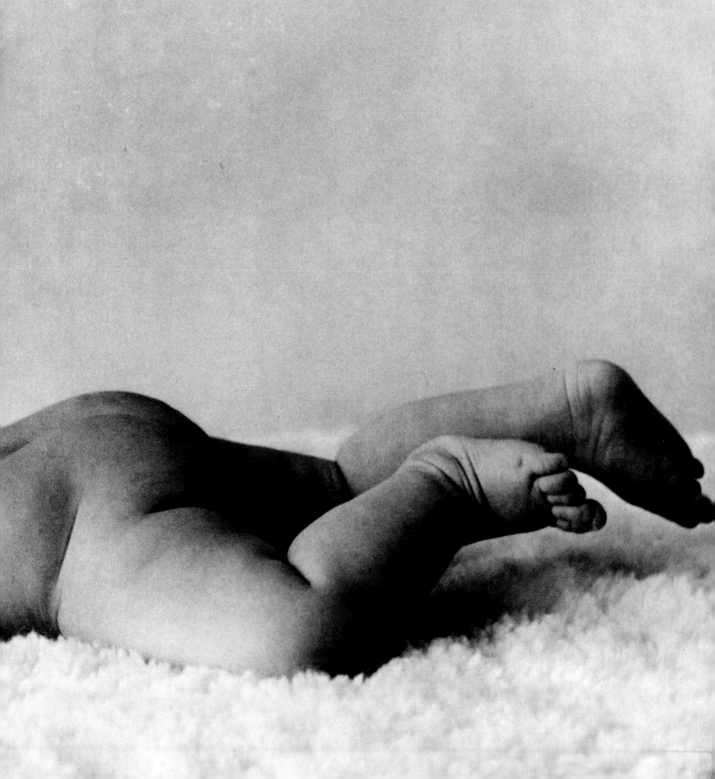

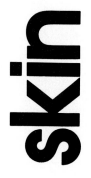

skin

The daily essentials

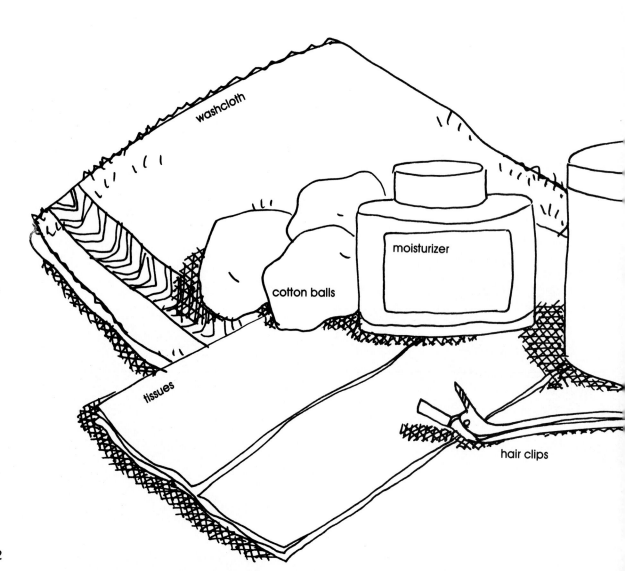

washcloth

cotton balls

moisturizer

tissues

hair clips

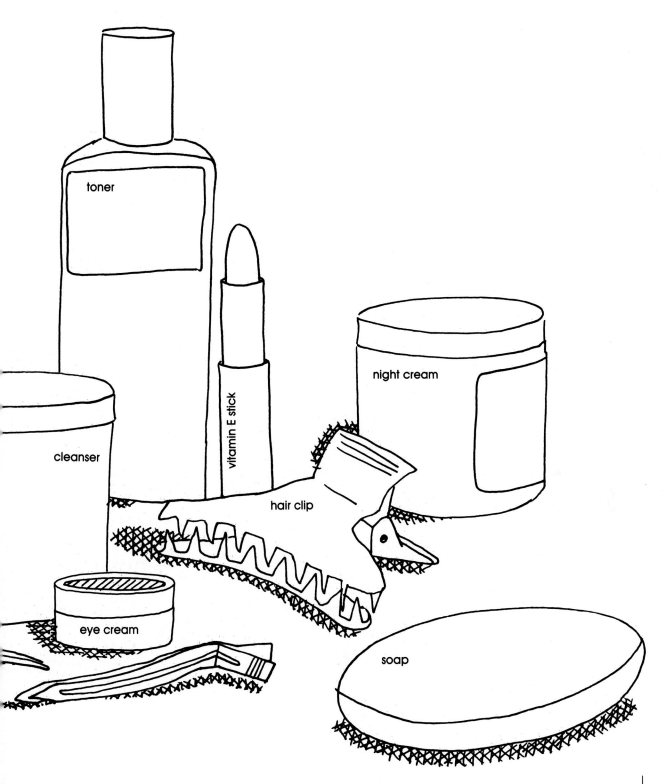

toner

vitamin E stick

cleanser

night cream

hair clip

eye cream

soap

23

skin

Each of us is born with a totally individual skin that is every bit as unique as our fingerprints. If we are lucky, we are taught when we are very young how best to care for it without fuss; but better late than never. Skin changes, reflects, protects and works a full twenty four hour day. It's often exposed to extreme temperatures—burning heat, biting cold—and the soot and grime of our daily lives. Get to know your skin intimately. Treat it like your best friend: gently, because the skin is sensitive; consistently, because crash programs don't work; patiently, because it'll pay off in the long run.

SPECIAL USES (ALL SKINS)

Photography

Cake foundation, damp sponge applied/blended
Dry cake makeup, wet sponge applied/blended
Stick makeup, oil based, dry sponge blended

Enemies of the skin

Alcohol straight from the bottle
Soapy residue
Deodorant soaps
Detergent soaps

SKIN PRODUCTS

PRODUCT	DRY SKIN	NORMAL SKIN	OILY SKIN
SOAPS	Superfatted Unscented Baby Liquid	Superfatted Clear/glycerine Unscented Designer/imported Baby Liquid	Clear Unscented Baby
CLEANSERS	Lotion *(rinse off)* Lotion *(tissue off)* Cream *(rinse or tissue off)*	Lotion *(rinse or tissue off)* Cream *(rinse or tissue off)*	Grainy—*only once weekly on oily areas*
FRESHENERS	Mild only	Mild Medium strength	Strong
MOISTURIZERS	Cream *(heavy)* Lotion *(heavy)*	Cream *(light)* Lotion *(light)*	Cream *(light)* Lotion *(light)* *(Used only on dry areas)*
NEUTRALIZERS	Lavender *(sallow skin)* Aqua *(ruddy skin)* Both in lotion form	Lavender *(sallow skin)* Aqua *(ruddy skin)* Both in lotion form	Lavender *(sallow skin)* Aqua *(ruddy skin)* Both in lotion form
FOUNDATIONS	Liquid *(water based)* Emulsion *(water based)* Liquid *(oil based)* Cream *(water based)* Cream *(oil based)* Cake	Liquid *(water based)* Emulsion *(water based)* Cream *(water based— soufflé)* Cake cream/dry	Liquid *(water based)* Liquid *powder (shake before using)* Oil free Oil blotting Oil control
NIGHT CREAMS	The best: Crisco from the can	Crisco from the can	Crisco on eye area only

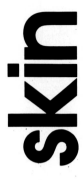

SKIN TYPE	PM	AM
NORMAL Dermatologists define normal skin as one that can adjust to change quickly. A blemish or spot may flare up occasionally, but on the whole it stays clear and is untemperamental.	Keeping eyes closed, wipe oil soaked pad across and over the eye area; rinse with cloth and hot water five or six times. Then scrub with superfatted soap and water, making a lather. Rinse face with cloth under running water at least fifteen times or until all residue of soap is gone. Squeeze out the cloth. Semidry the face with a patting motion. Immediately apply moisturizer to every millimeter of slightly damp face. Blend in well with ring finger, the gentlest one.	Splash with lukewarm water. Pat semidry. Apply moisturizer.
DRY Dry skin tends to be taut and transparent, and is quick to show lack of moisture by developing fine lines. This type of skin needs particularly gentle care both in cleansing and in lubricating. The trick to correct treatment is to be *gentle* (thus avoiding broken capillaries) and to moisturize consistently.	Cleanse, rinse and moisturize exactly as above. For additional moisture, apply an eye cream or lubricating stick on drier areas around the eyes, the laugh lines and wherever else you need it.	Splash and moisturize as above.
OILY Cleansing is of the utmost importance to this skin type as it tends to absorb pollution, dirt and makeup. It is especially susceptible to skin eruptions. One long run benefit of oily skin is that it is less likely to wrinkle and stays younger looking longer.	Cleanse and rinse as for normal skin. Then encircle the eye area with a thin layer of moisturizer, lubricating stick or eye cream.	Cleanse, rinse and moisturize exactly as you did at night. This is the only skin type that needs two washings within twenty four hours.

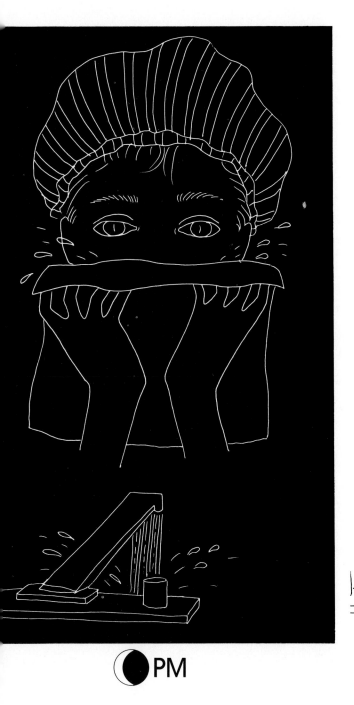

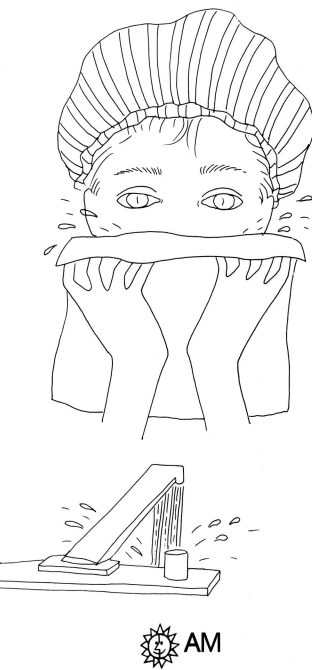

PM

AM

27

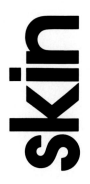

skin

CLEANSING AND MAINTENANCE: A RELIGIOUS EXPERIENCE

Cleansing

Makeup needs to be taken off as carefully as it is put on, so washing with soap and water is one of the first routines that Beauty Checkers teaches.

First, wet your skin with warm to hot running water. (*Never* simply put soap to a dry face). Then, using a superfatted soap, lather well—up into the hairline, down into the neck, back into the ears, just avoiding the eye area.

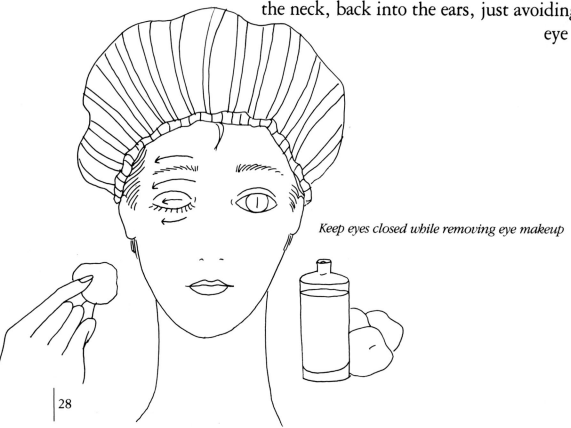

Keep eyes closed while removing eye makeup

28

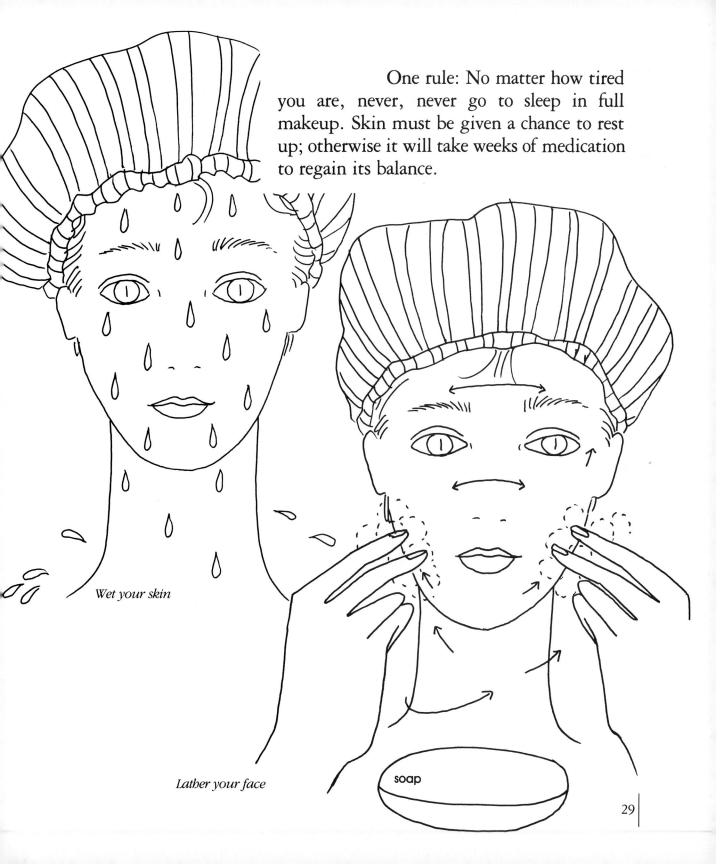

One rule: No matter how tired you are, never, never go to sleep in full makeup. Skin must be given a chance to rest up; otherwise it will take weeks of medication to regain its balance.

Wet your skin

Lather your face

soap

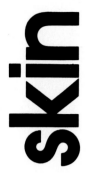

Rinsing

Rinsing is of the utmost importance because it helps counteract the drying ingredients that are a part of every soap. And we have found that water, inexpensive though it may be, is an excellent substitute for toners, fresheners and astringents.

Fifteen to twenty rinses—it only takes an extra minute—are needed to be sure that every smidgen of soapy residue has vanished. You will feel wonderful when your face is squeaky clean.

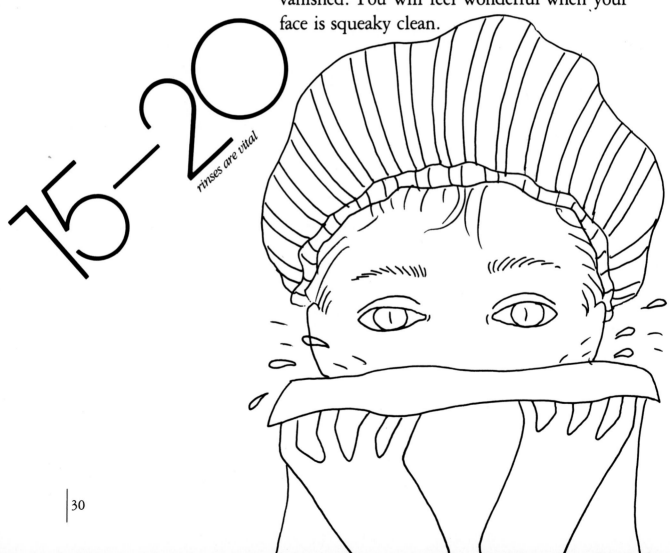

15-20 *rinses are vital*

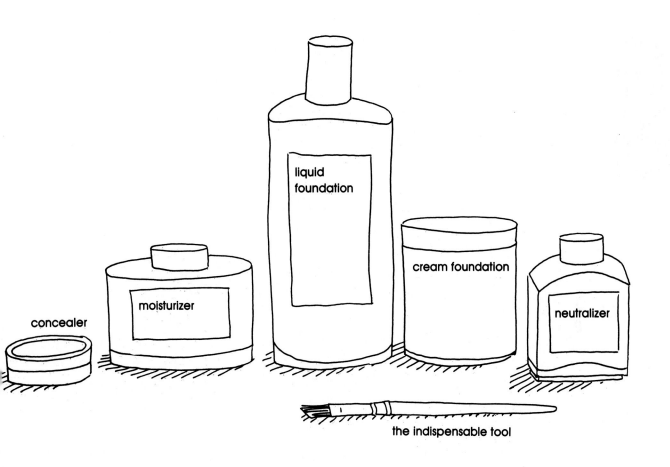

concealer

moisturizer

liquid
foundation

cream foundation

neutralizer

the indispensable tool

MAINTENANCE

Think of your skin tending as a kind of insurance plan. The better you take care of your complexion now, the less help you'll need later on.

Moisturizer

No matter what *anyone* tells you, after puberty one item that everyone must use daily is a moisturizer—not only as a lubricant, but also as protection against pollution. A mois-

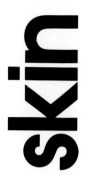

skin

turizer is actually a shield to prevent your own facial moisture from evaporating too quickly. Many women think adding moisture to an oil-producing face is like bringing a pipeline into Kuwait, but in fact, every living face, oily or not, needs lubrication in certain areas, particularly the eye area and neck.

If whatever brand you use feels right, be loyal to it. Of course, you may find that you need a heavier moisturizer in the winter or in cold climates than you do in the summer or in a more humid climate. If so, don't hesitate to switch. It is definitely worth remembering (if you're not satisfied with what you're using and plan to switch brands) that expense isn't always the best measure of a good moisturizer. In today's burgeoning marketplace you have endless choices in a wide price range (see Skin Products Chart, p. 25 at the beginning of this chapter).

Q. *What is a night cream?*
A. A heavier type of moisturizer: Usually in cream form, too gooey to wear under makeup, but good for your sleeping face. Crisco, which is pure vegetable shortening, makes an excellent night cream. No one has ever broken out from it.

Q. *I'm under thirty. Do I need a night cream?*
A. Absolutely. We recommend that you anoint your squeaky clean face with a thin film of Crisco.

Crisco
makes an excellent
night cream

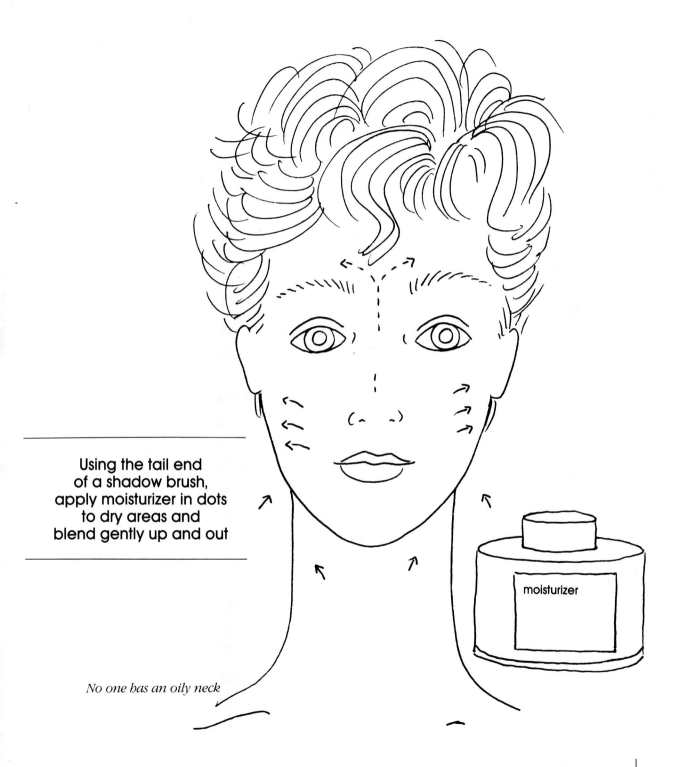

Using the tail end
of a shadow brush,
apply moisturizer in dots
to dry areas and
blend gently up and out

No one has an oily neck

moisturizer

skin

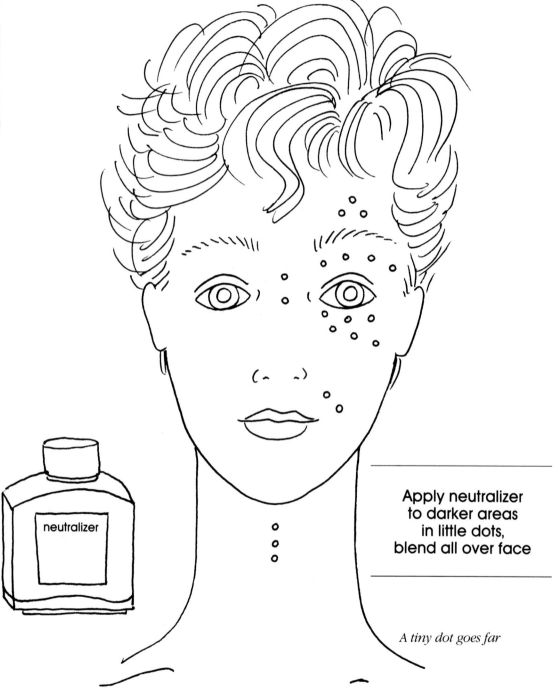

neutralizer

Apply neutralizer
to darker areas
in little dots,
blend all over face

A tiny dot goes far

SKIN TONE: RUDDY OR SALLOW—nature's flip of the coin

Heredity, age and pollution ensure that no one has an even or perfect skin tone. Some of us are pale—sallow, yellow or greenish, especially after we lose a tan. Smoking, drinking, drugs, improper diet, tension and lack of exercise all aggravate the sickly pallor. Others of us are florid, blotchy or plagued with little red broken capillaries. This condition is aggravated by drinking, tension and extremes of temperature.

Each of us falls into one category or another. Foundation can't cover it all without help, so we need a primer (much like the one a painter uses), to even out the skin tone and act as a first coat so that the foundation can do its work more effectively. This primer is what we call a "neutralizer." Lavender is for sallow complexions; aqua for florid ones. Neutralizer is applied over moisturizer in tiny dots, wherever your color is uneven, usually all over the face. It is always used *lightly* under foundation.

Q. *Can I wear neutralizer without a foundation?*

A. No. You'll look like a corpse.

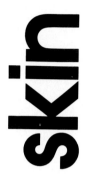

skin

**Always use
half the foundation
you think
you'll need**

Q. *I never wear foundation. Do I really need it?*

A. Yes, of course, if you want your skin to look finished. Beauty Checkers doesn't mean you should lay it on with a trowel and wind up looking like a 1930s movie vamp. *Light-handed* but effective is the key.

Always put foundation on in the best possible light—ideally in front of a makeup mirror or a window. Always use half the foundation you think you'll need (it's easier to add than to take away). As you blend it in, be gentle to your face. Don't ever rub or pound. You're handling your precious skin, not making a loaf of bread! You'll instantly be aware of the fringe benefits of your moisturizer, as it helps foundation to cling like a second skin. Every motion should be up and out—and GENTLE.

A foundation will camouflage minor imperfections and minimize natural skin flaws. The resulting smoothness will cause your features to be displayed to their full advantage. This is why when you only apply eye makeup or blusher or lip color, *it doesn't help* . . . if you're over eighteen.

Q. *Where should I look for the right foundation?*

A. Head for your local drugstore, variety store, department store or cosmetics boutique . . . preferably during the day so you can see the color in natural light.

Q. *What do I do when I get to the cosmetics counter?*

A. You must learn to try on foundation for color and fit much the way you try on shoes before buying. Wearing moisturizer and neutralizer but no foundation, test the color on your face—not on your underwrist, which is about ten shades lighter than your face. When you've found your shade, buy it, take it home and use it daily—not only for special occasions.

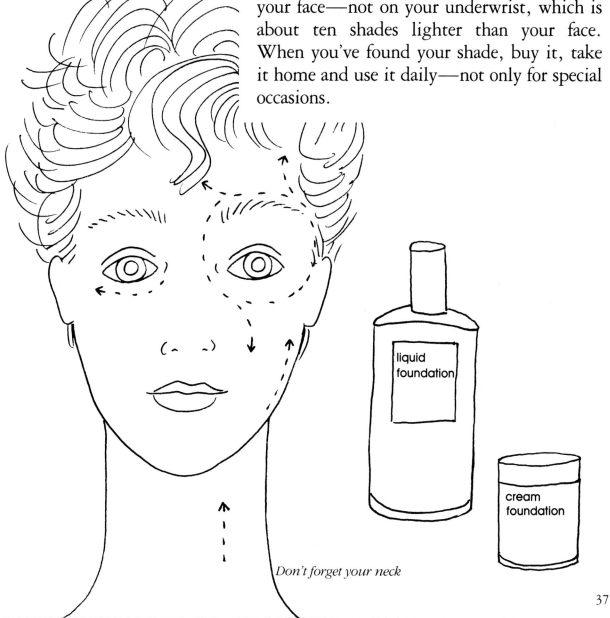

Don't forget your neck

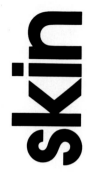

skin

NUISANCES REDUCED TO SIZE

Minor eruptions

So you've got a blemish just before your fourth and deciding interview, when you want to look perfect. *What to do?*

1. Don't panic. You notice it more than anyone else.
2. Don't squeeze or fiddle.
3. Hide it.

How to camouflage

1. Moisturize
2. Neutralize
3. Apply foundation and . . .
4. A flesh colored concealer, matching your skin tone as closely as possible. Pat it directly on the blemish, over the foundation. Apply a dab of loose translucent powder with a cotton swab, directly on top of the concealer. Let it sit while you complete your makeup. Then brush it off gently with a cotton ball.

Freckles

We find freckles charming and think it is sad to cover them up completely. (Then again, all of us haven't lived a lifetime with freckles.) Let's compromise. Follow your usual moistur-

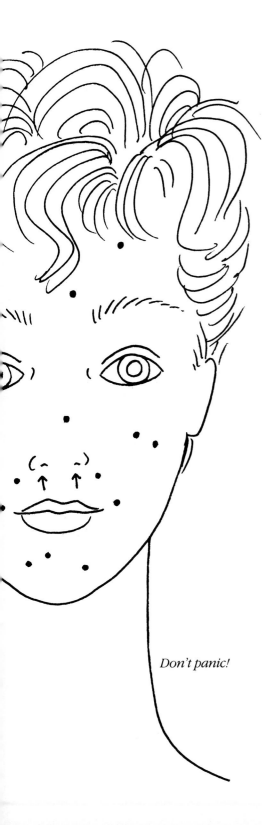

Don't panic!

izer, neutralizer, foundation routine. Making up your eyes, lips and cheeks will automatically make your freckles less prominent by turning attention away from them.

KEEP OUT OF THE SUN!

If you're hell bent on a tan, at least wear a sunblock and a large hat. Freckles proliferate in the sun.

If you apply sunblock in the morning before exposure and then swim, run around, play ball, perspire and don't reapply the sunblock frequently, *you will burn.*

Facial hair

In our culture, it is completely taboo, so most urban centers offer the following options for its removal. First and foremost:

Go to a professional ...

even if it means scrimping on something else.

Waxing: This is painful, expensive and has to be repeated every few weeks, depending on how fast your hairs grow.

Electrolysis: More painful, more expensive, but usually permanent.

Plucking: If you must do it yourself: PLEASE, only with an impeccable, sanitary, back into its own case tweezer. In sunlight, with a magnifying mirror. *Bonne chance.*

Depilatories: Sometimes work.

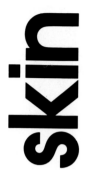

skin

Bleaching: Good for the first peach fuzz on young skin. (It is close to what the sun does.) But anything more will oxidize when bleached, often turning orange.

Shaving: Women should never shave their faces. Period.

TODAY'S SKIN— TOMORROW'S WRINKLE

The aging process begins the day we are born, but the extent to which it affects our skin is up to us. Skin is like a bank account—you can't keep withdrawing without daily deposits and expect a normal balance in middle age. It's a question of awareness, self-esteem and lifestyle.

Usual causes of wrinkling

Heredity: The most significant. If you resemble your parents, chances are you'll wrinkle like them. But with today's know how, it will happen ten years later—if you make a consistent effort.

Sun and weather: This can be partially controlled with the right protection, which is available in every price range.

Tension: This will deepen every line, and eventually cement them in. Become aware of the areas of tension in your face:

forehead, eyes, mouth. Consciously relax them, whenever you feel tense.

Illness: This really takes its toll, even if it's only a head cold. The culprit is dehydration. Drink gallons of fluids and double your normal vitamin intake (A, D and E are the skin vitamins). Always check with your doctor first.

If there is high fever or shock to the system resulting from medication or anesthesia, you should slather on plenty of heavy duty moisturizer (i.e., Crisco from the can)—even if it's the last thing you feel like doing. A week later you'll thank us.

Routine self abuse (smoking, drugs, alcohol, etc.): Yes, it sounds menacing, but yours is the only skin you'll ever have. (Alcohol remains in the system for seventy two hours after intake.)

If your wrinkles, crow's feet, baggy undereyes, droopy overlids or jowls are unbearable to live with, have them corrected with cosmetic surgery. We don't mean to take this very expensive and serious subject lightly . . . but be aware that in today's world it is a service that is readily available. Check with your family doctor—or with the AMA—for reference. Miracles are performed everyday—and as a morale booster, it's longer lasting than a weekend in Paris with your lover.

cheeks

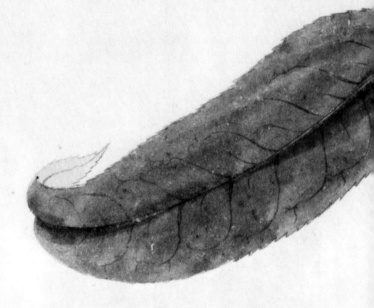

Peaches 'n'
cream

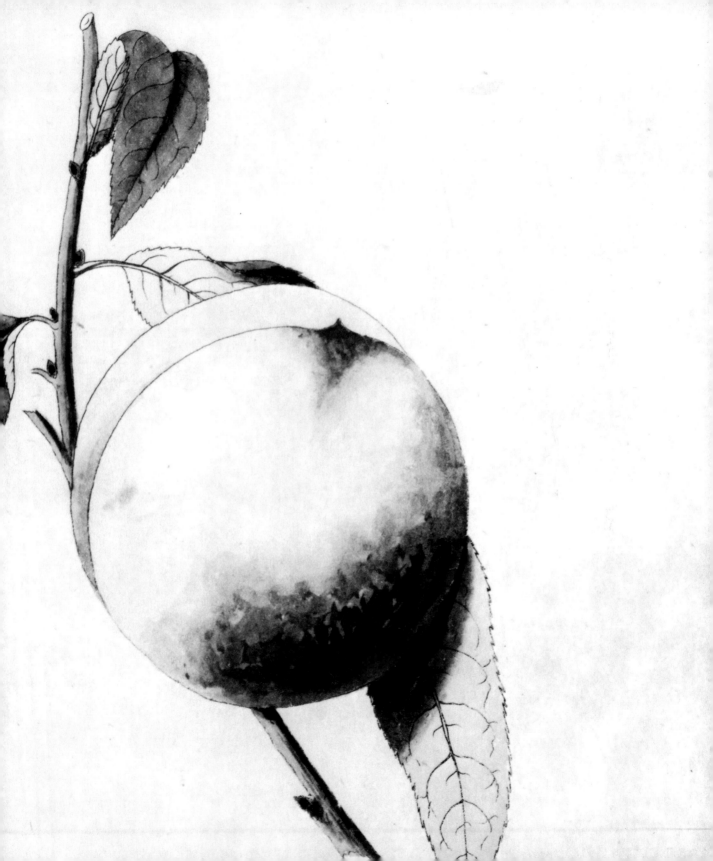

cheeks

Ninety nine out of a hundred women don't know how—and where—to apply rouge.

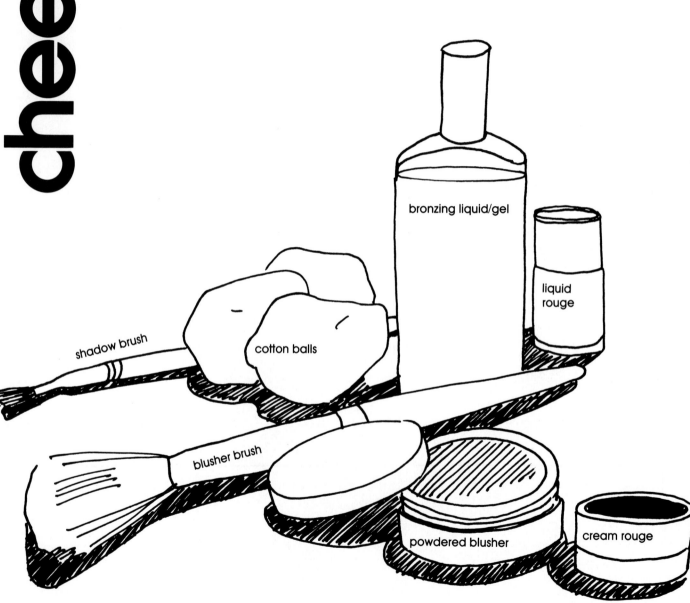

shadow brush

cotton balls

bronzing liquid/gel

liquid rouge

blusher brush

powdered blusher

cream rouge

At Beauty Checkers, women are forever asking if their blusher is the right color, but very few ask *where* the color should go. And in our experience the average woman hasn't a clue about this. All she knows is that she wants to "glow." Looking like an Indian in full war paint isn't necessarily the best way to achieve this effect, however.

CHEEK PRODUCTS

PRODUCT	SALLOW SKIN	FLORID SKIN	DARK SKIN
CREAM ROUGE In flat container or stick form	PEACH CORAL PLUM RED	PINK MELON Avoid brown, plum, bright red	BRICK, BURGUNDY BRIGHT: PINK ORANGE RED Avoid pastels and brown
LIQUID ROUGE OR GEL	*As above*	NO	BRONZY GOLD
POWDERED BLUSHER	PEACH MELON GOLD FROST RED Avoid anything muddy looking	PINK MELON Avoid brown, plum, red	MULBERRY BRICK BRIGHT: PINK ORANGE RED Avoid pastels or muddy colors
LOOSE POWDERED ROUGE (Henna)	FOR SUMMER ONLY (Looks awful on pasty winter faces)	NO	MADE FOR YOU

cheeks

CONTOURING/ SHADING— A MISGUIDED NOTION

Beauty Checkers—reinforced by years of visually painful experience—dislikes "contouring" and wants to dispel the myth that it creates high cheekbones and angles the face. How the idea of "contouring" or "shading" reached such heights of popularity (culminating in the skeletal face of the 1960s) is something of a mystery. Even for photography, the right lighting will throw cheekbones into relief as no "shading" ever could. "Contouring" for the average woman *does not work*. Usually it looks like five o'clock shadow—at best, like a slightly dirty face. For everyday makeup, it is a total waste of time and effort.

Forget about contouring/shading altogether—and concentrate on looking pretty instead.

ROUGE AND BLUSHER— A STROKE OF COLOR

You have now prepared your face as though it were a canvas. Everything you've done up to this point has been basic. Now it's time for color. But where should the rouge go?

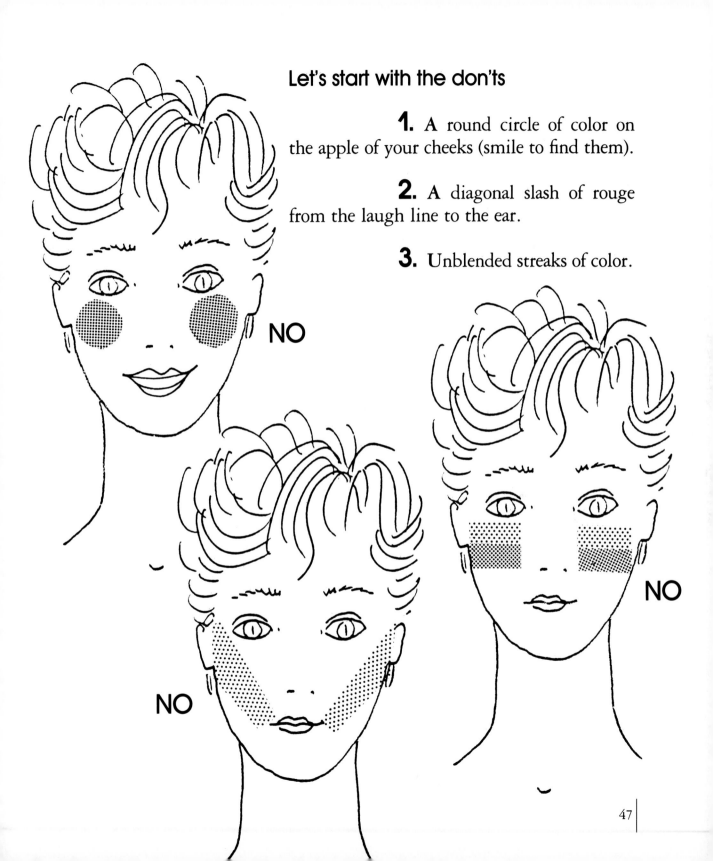

Let's start with the don'ts

1. A round circle of color on the apple of your cheeks (smile to find them).

2. A diagonal slash of rouge from the laugh line to the ear.

3. Unblended streaks of color.

NO

NO

NO

47

cheeks

And now the do's

1. Everyone's face is lopsided. To get the right perspective, you must look straight ahead into the mirror.

2. Suck in your cheeks; dot cream (or liquid) rouge along your cheekbone in a crescent shape, starting at the temple (see diagram). With your ring finger, for the right pressure, gently blend it up and out into the hairline.

Cream rouge— the simplest to control

Blending *must* be gentle—because the action of pressing down on your skin always brings the blood up to the surface. When this subsides, you'll look paler. Don't be surprised— it's normal. Why? Years of pillow pressure cause the skin to reject color. The side of the face you sleep on fades faster than the other.

Reapply the rouge till you get the desired evenness. You may have to put three applications on the fading side before it will match the other.

The big advantage of cream rouge is that if you make a mistake you can easily tissue it off (gently) and start over.

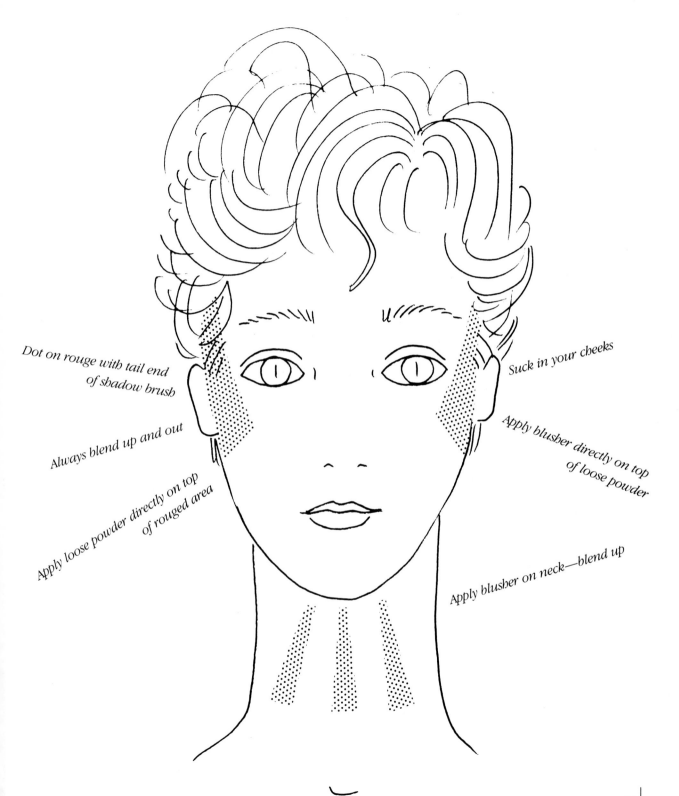

Dot on rouge with tail end
of shadow brush

Always blend up and out

Apply loose powder directly on top
of rouged area

Suck in your cheeks

Apply blusher directly on top
of loose powder

Apply blusher on neck—blend up

cheeks

Liquid rouge

Liquid rouges are trickier since they dry immediately upon contact. Once dotted on, liquid rouge must be blended instantly—pause to pick up the phone or the baby and the delay between dotting and blending will leave you with red spots sitting on your face like measles. This means you'll have to clean your face and start the makeup all over again.

Always check rouge color by daylight after you put it on in the morning. You may look like Camille in the bathroom mirror and like Pocahontas in the light of your bedroom window. Make the necessary adjustments.

Gels

Face color in a gel base tends to contain alcohol, so it dries quickly on the skin. This means that before you use it you must know exactly where you want it to go—and be sure to apply moisturizer first.

Gels generally come in a tube. They should not go all over the face, but should be applied high up on the cheekbones, on the neck, forehead, temples and chin—for a "sunkissed" effect. Gel is a great makeup for winter white legs. *Warning:* It does have a tendency to stick to blemishes and turn them redder . . . use with body balm.

A delay between dotting
and blending will
leave you with red spots
sitting on your face
like measles

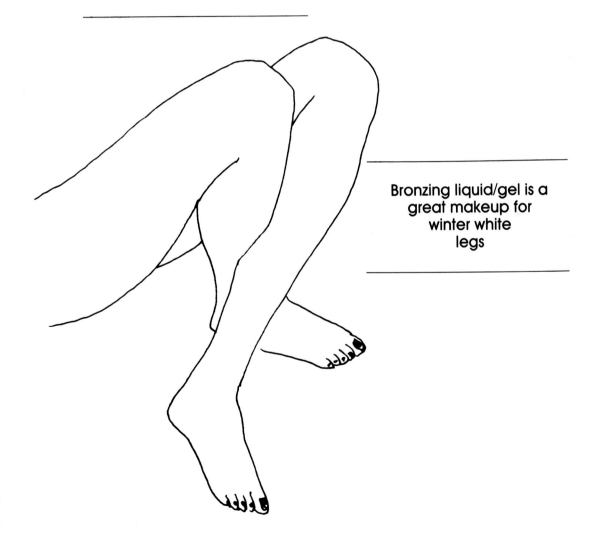

Bronzing liquid/gel is a
great makeup for
winter white
legs

cheeks

Powdered blusher

This is best used in *conjunction* with cream rouge, not *instead* of it. The whole trick is to apply powdered blusher over a bed of loose powder. Apply with a cotton ball—that you instantly dispose of—and blend together with a generous brush (*not* the same one you will use for your powder, a medium size version.) If you apply cream rouge, a layer of powder directly over it and blusher on top of that, *you will not fade for three or four hours.*

The whole trick is
to apply powdered blusher
over a bed
of loose powder

cream rouge +

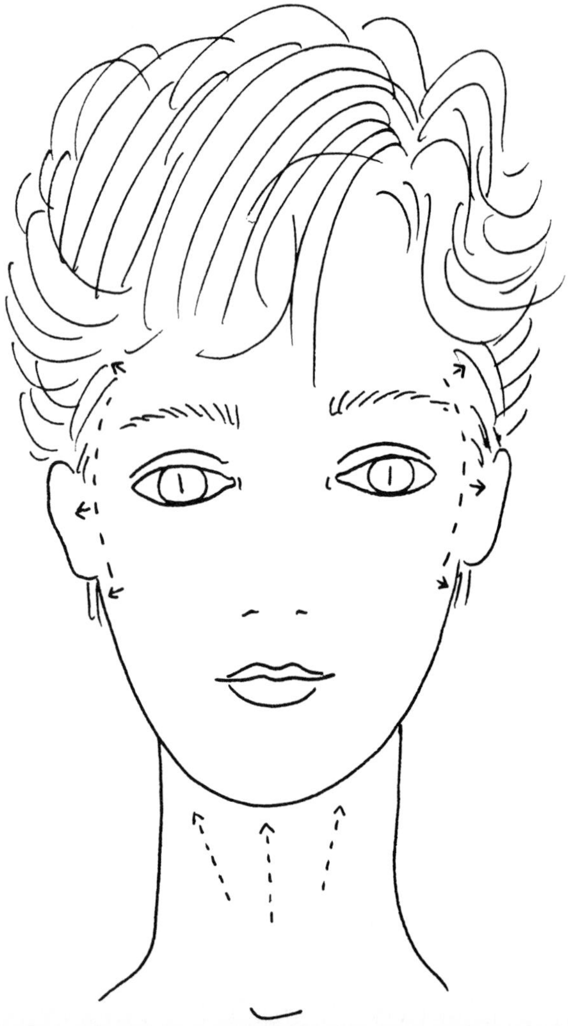

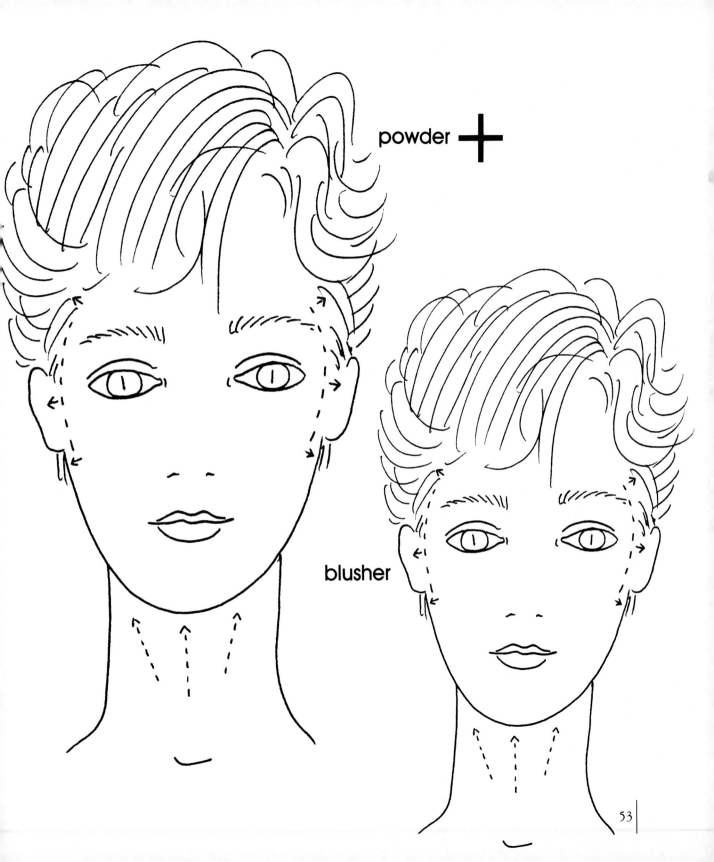

powder **+**

blusher

cheeks

LOOSE POWDER— THE FORGOTTEN COSMETIC

Do you remember loose powder?

You should—it's made a big comeback in the last decade. In fact, it has now shaken off the stigma of being for "mothers only." It never was, of course—professional makeup people never stopped using it. Unfortunately, the mistaken impression that it "closes your pores" and "dries your skin" persists. This is simply not so.

We have introduced thousands of women to loose powder, and they have become total devotees. Of course, we don't recommend hopping out of bed and diving right into your powder box—but after your face has been made up, the powder will never touch your skin. Instead it rests on the surface like a fine veil, hiding a multitude of sins. Therefore, it neither clogs your pores nor dries your skin—and remember, only the very young look good with a shine.

Apply your loose powder lightly all over with a fresh cotton ball . . . blend with a clean and generous brush. Concentrate on the T zone—chin, nose, forehead —and *don't forget your neck.*

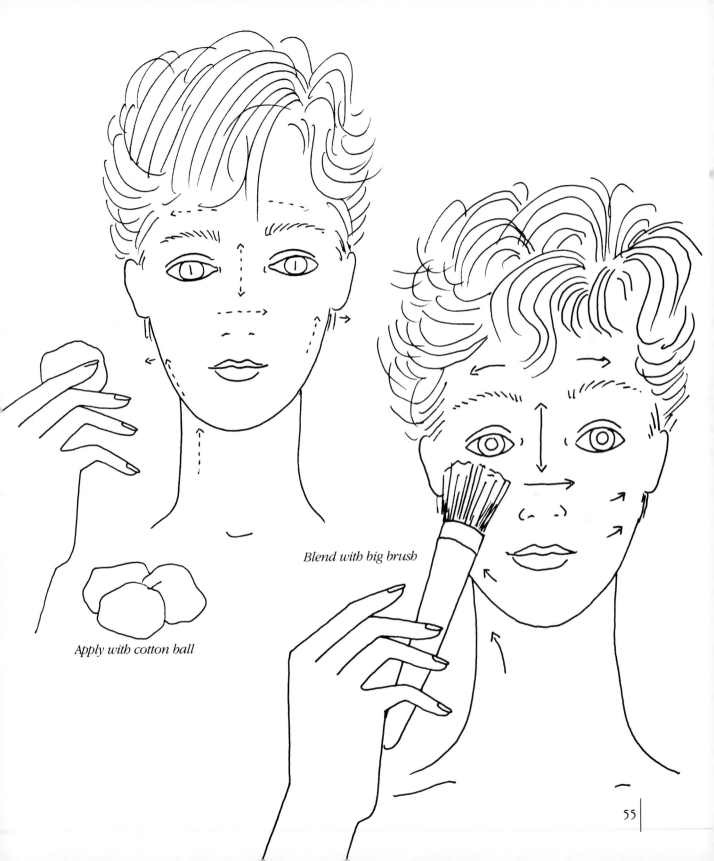

Apply with cotton ball

Blend with big brush

cheeks

Use translucent powder only; it's colorless and won't turn

Use a fresh cotton ball to apply powder

Basic powder rules

1. Webster's definition of "translucent" is "admitting and diffusing light so that objects beyond cannot be clearly distinguished." Our sentiments exactly. Face powder is the ultimate flatterer. Use translucent powder only—it's colorless and won't turn.

2. Use only a fresh cotton ball to apply powder; throw out used ones as soon as you've finished the makeup—for total cleanliness. That's at home. Powder puffs are great for compacts, but *change* them.

3. All brushes, including your powder brush, must be immaculate. Wash brushes at least once a week. Use mild soap in tepid running water as washing a brush in alcohol will make it sticky and hard.

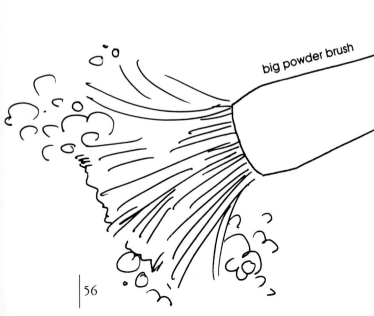

big powder brush

All brushes, including your powder brush, must be immaculate

Touch up rules

No makeup
lasts
all day

Powder will help your makeup remain stable much longer—it holds back body heat. NO MAKEUP LASTS ALL DAY. Don't expect it to—and don't be disappointed when it fades. Every three or four hours, you'll need to touch up. Carry with you in a plastic sandwich bag:

- *tissues*
- *cotton swabs*
- *loose or pressed powder*
- *blusher*
- *cotton balls*
- *mirror*

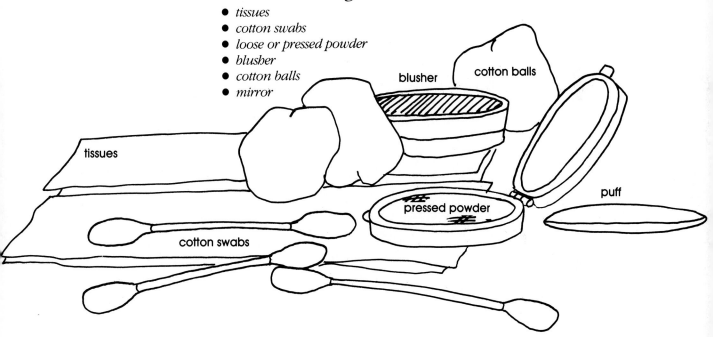

tissues

blusher

cotton balls

puff

pressed powder

cotton swabs

In a powder room wipe the T zone gently with the tissue wrapped around your forefinger (*not* scrunched up into a ball). Smooth out the eye area gently with a cotton ball. Don't forget to dab a bit of color on the sides of your neck and blend. The whole procedure, including washing your hands and combing your hair, will take three minutes.

57

eyes

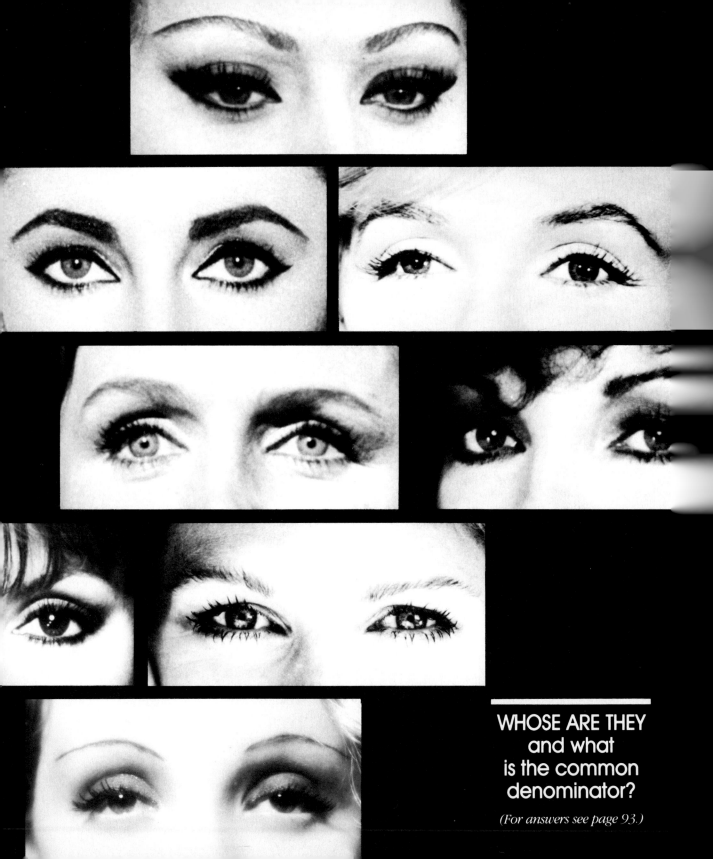

WHOSE ARE THEY
and what
is the common
denominator?

(For answers see page 93.)

eyes

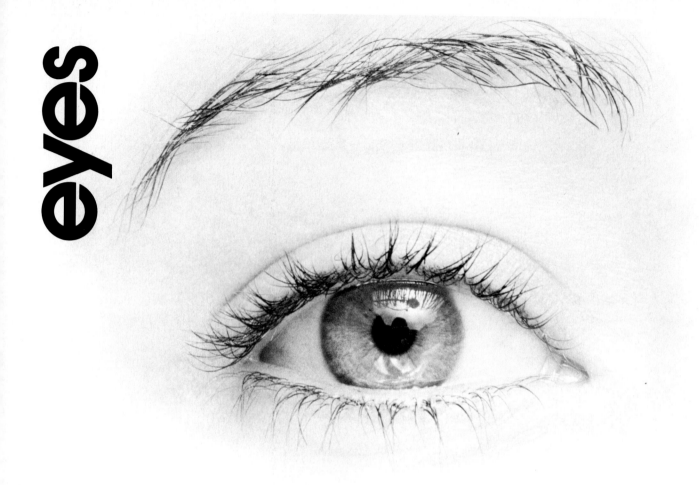

Before

Most women take for granted that their eyes are their best feature. Billions of dollars are spent annually on eye makeup and the cosmetic companies, knowing this, constantly introduce new colors and improve their eye products. In spite of this, women tend to be amazingly reluctant to change the way they do their eyes; they cling to what is familiar.

Brown shadow and black liner, the signature of the 1950s and 1960s, die

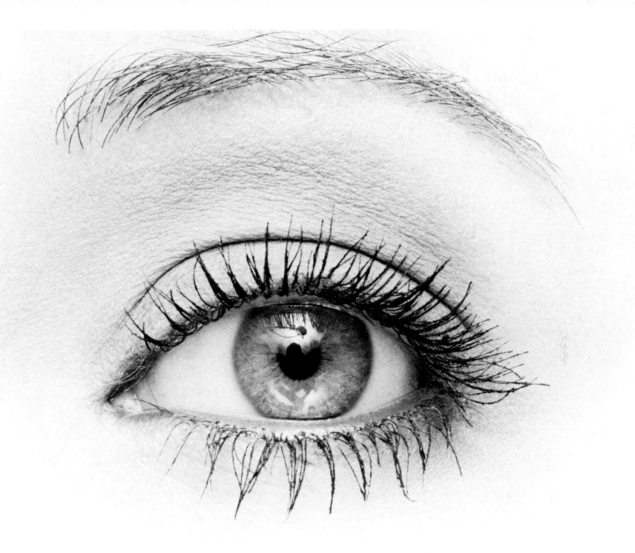

After

hard. And yet old fashioned eye makeup will instantly date an otherwise beautifully madeup face.

Eye makeup should be used to enhance your eyes. The products themselves must never be noticed. The key to good eye makeup is "balance," both in the way it is blended and in the amount applied.

Nothing is as aging as eye makeup that enters a room before its owner.

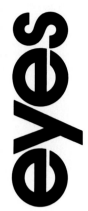

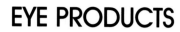

PRODUCT	AM EYE	PM EYE	EXTRA SPECIAL EYE	MATURE EYE
CONCEALER: *Cream, liquid, or stick form*	**YES:** Any form	**YES:** Any form	**YES:** Any form	**YES:** Cream or liquid
LOOSE POWDER *for whole eyelid*	YES	YES	YES	YES
POWDERED EYESHADOW	YES	YES	YES	NO
CREAM *or liquid eyeshadow*	NO	YES	YES	**YES:** Liquid and only in flesh tones
EYESHADOW PENCILS *(fat and creamy)*	YES	YES	YES	NO
THIN LINER EYE PENCIL	YES	YES	YES	**BLUE ONLY:** In strategic areas
LIQUID LINER	NO	NO	**NO:** Resist!	NO
LASH CURLER	NO	YES	YES	NO
MASCARA	YES	YES	YES	**YES:** On outer corner only
COTTON SWABS, *shadow brush, comb/brush, sharpener*	YES	YES	YES	YES

For your eyes only

*Clean, sharpened
and at the ready—
just use them,
cover them
and put them back.
The three eyeshadows
should complement
each other*

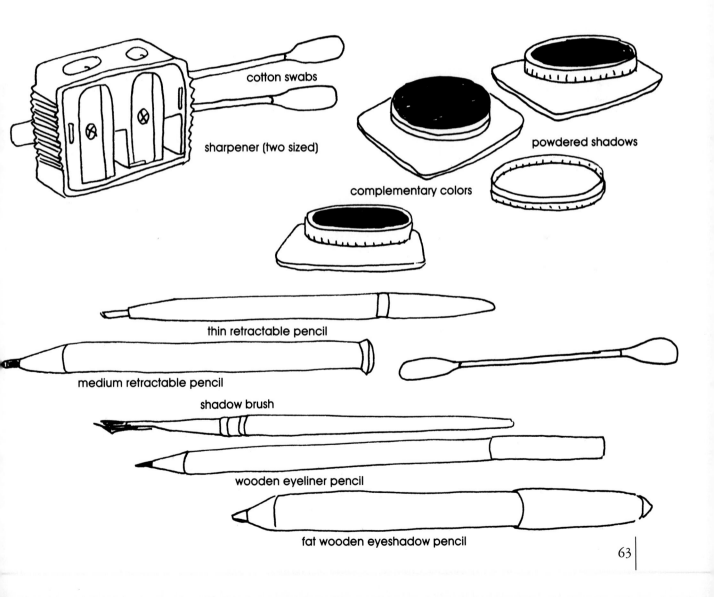

cotton swabs

sharpener (two sized)

complementary colors

powdered shadows

thin retractable pencil

medium retractable pencil

shadow brush

wooden eyeliner pencil

fat wooden eyeshadow pencil

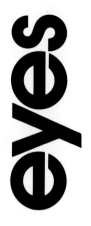

eyes

DARK CIRCLES—
FOR PANDAS ONLY

Nearly everyone has darkness around the eyes. The darkness is over the eye as well as under and especially in the corners. Also, the eyelid is often darker and more discolored than the undereye area. There are many causes for the darkness, which actually bears little relation to a person's age. Young people are as prone to dark circles as older ones.

Causes include heredity, smoking and other excesses, fatigue, illness, the wrong diet, lack of exercise and fresh air, stress, contact lenses and makeup residue.

Puffiness ("bags") under the eyes and of the eyelids are equally common; both can be caused by liquid retention (especially upon waking in the morning), allergies, smoking and other excesses, infection, irritation, heredity and steroids (such as cortisone). In older or middle age people, puffiness is often caused by herniated fat sacs under the skin or any of the above.

COPING WITH
CIRCLES AND PUFFINESS

First of all: Make sure that when you apply makeup to your face (moisturizer and/or vitamin E stick, neutralizer and foundation), you remember to include your eye area.

Lighten the tiny veins and natural darkness around the eye. This is done with a "darkness concealer," which can be in soft stick, paste, liquid or cream form. Concealer is applied in tiny dots wherever needed,

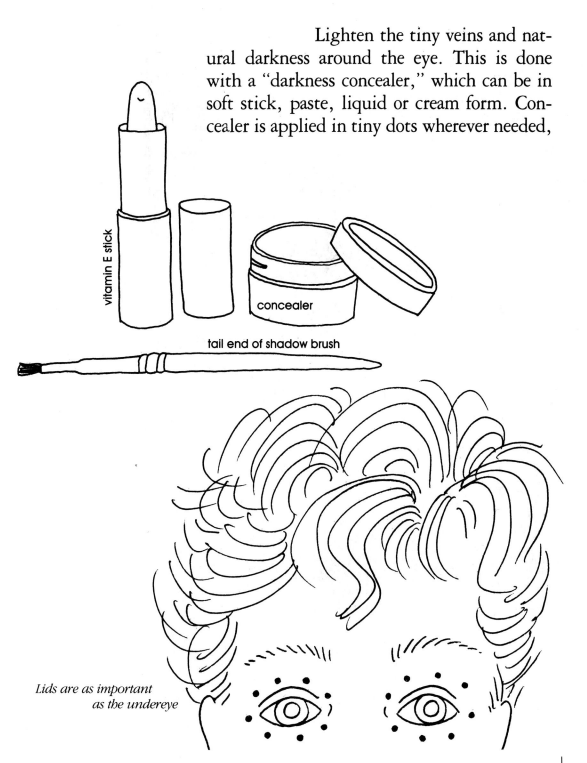

vitamin E stick

concealer

tail end of shadow brush

Lids are as important as the undereye

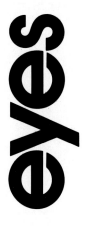

and is thoroughly blended to avoid demarcation lines. Since the eye area has no oil glands, you may have to add a little moisturizer or vitamin E stick for extra blendability. Darkness concealer should be lighter than your foundation—and always applied over it. A darker color over a lighter one defeats its own purpose. Darkness concealer works well on blemishes and laugh lines, too.

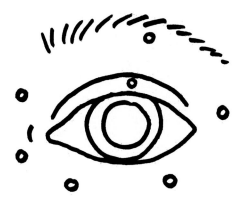

**Darkness concealer
should always be lighter
than your foundation,
and always
applied over it**

OPTICAL ILLUSIONS

Before reading this section, determine the shape of your eye. Then concentrate on the eye makeup that applies specifically to you by comparing it to our sketches.

Always powder all over eyelid using small brush end.

☐ Small eyes   ☐ Wide set eyes

☐ Round eyes   ☐ Bland eyes

☐ Droopy lids   ☐ Almond or Oriental eyes

☐ Deep set eyes   ☐ Crepey lids

☐ Narrow squinty eyes   ☐ Bulging or puffy eyes

☐ Close set eyes   ☐ Perfect eyes

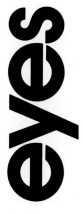

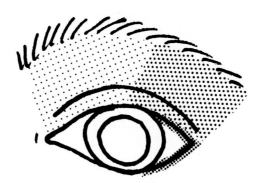

Small eyes

1. Ivory, yellow, eggnog or other pastel (not white) shadow on inner corner of eye—extend up to midbrow and cover whole inner half of eye.
2. Darker color (plum, light gray, medium blue, dark green) on outer half of eye; blend together with light shadow at mideye. Extend darker color out beyond brow. Blend well.
3. Highlighter (pink, yellow) over end of brow.
4. Little dots of color (thin blue or gray pencil) at base of upper outer lashes . . . carry dots around corner of eye and then draw thin blue or gray line directly beneath lower lashes, stopping where your lashes stop.
5. Same thin pencil on lower inner rim of eye, to make whites give the illusion of size.
6. *Black* mascara only on upper outer corners and lower outer corners.

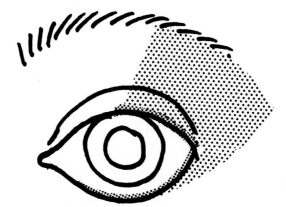

Round eyes

1. Light pastel shadow (eggnog, pink, nude, etc.) on entire eyelid, from inner corner next to nose, right up into brow and out to the end.
2. Medium dark shadow (plum, light gray, medium blue, dark green) on outer corner of eye, across outer third of upper lid. Carry a smidgen of shadow around corner of eye.
Blend up and out.
3. Thin, medium shade pencil line at base of upper and lower lashes. Work on outer third of eye only.
4. With thin blue pencil, line inner rim of eye, upper and lower. Go a third of the way in from outer corner.
5. Mascara on upper and lower lashes.

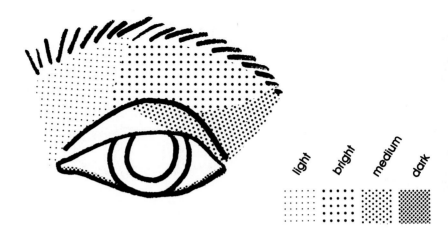

light bright medium dark

Droopy lids

1. Darken droopy area with medium shade (plum, light gray, medium blue, dark green). Be sure colors are well blended, and avoid brown or taupe—they will make you look tired.
2. Lighten the rest of the entire lid. The area just beneath the eyebrow, near the nose, should be especially lightened. Use matte ivory, eggnog, soft pastels; not white, as the contrast will be too great.
3. Line bottom inner rim of eye with soft blue, light purple or gray pencil.
4. No line outside the eye is necessary.
5. Black mascara on inner lashes only; lower as well as upper.

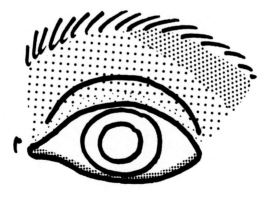

Deep set eyes

1. Light pastel shadow over entire eyelid (eggnog, ivory, yellow, pink), from inner corner up to brow and out to end. Fill in and blend well.
2. Darken area directly under brow from midpoint to outer corner. Use medium shades (light gray, plum, medium blue, dark green) and blend well into lighter color.
3. Use brighter color (pink, brick, russet, lavender, blue, green) just behind lashes from corner to corner.
4. Line lower inner rim with a thin blue pencil.
5. Curl upper lashes and use plenty of mascara—top and bottom.

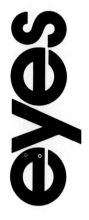

eyes

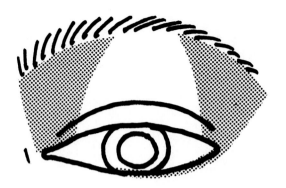

Narrow squinty eyes

1. Brighten entire lid—from inner corner to brow and out—with brick, yellow or your favorite blusher (yes, you can use it as a shadow). Blend well.
2. Darken *inner* corner up to brow using medium gray, gray-blue or dark green.
3. Darken outer corner up to brow bring-ing the same color around end of eye and under lower lashes. Get this shadow line as thin as possible.
4. Do not use pencil or liner.
5. Curl top lashes. Use black mascara liber-ally on top and bottom.

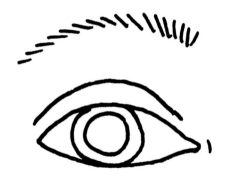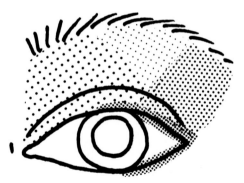

Close set eyes

1. Lighten entire eyelid with pastel color (eggnog, yellow, pink, etc.). Go from inner corner to brow and out.
2. Apply medium dark shadow (plum, light gray, medium blue, dark green) on outer corner of eye. Blend color up and out, al-most into rouge.
3. Apply a touch of your blusher to brow bone at outer corner.
4. Line outer upper edge as well as lower edge of eye with the same pencil. Blend well into lashes.
5. Brush mascara *outward,* almost horizon-tally.

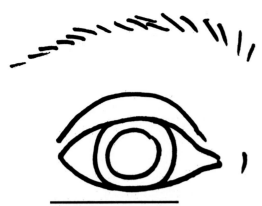
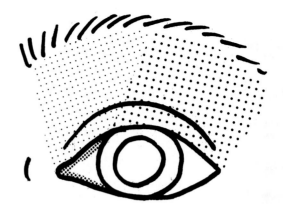

Wide set eyes

1. Brighten the inner third of eyelid (with russet, coral or pink shadow or blusher). Start next to nose, bringing color up and out.
2. Use a very light pastel (ivory or eggnog) on outer corner of eye, blending into brighter area.
3. Line inner rim of eye—upper and lower —with thin blue pencil, without going to the corner (otherwise your tear ducts will cause it to smudge).
4. Curl lashes and apply plenty of black mascara, giving inner lashes an extra coat. (Build them up with extra powder between coats.)

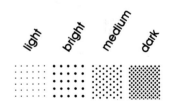

Bland eyes

These eyes are ripe for exploration. Buy yourself an inexpensive eyeshadow kit at your local variety store and play with it when you have a little time to yourself.
Try doing one eye in one set of colors and the other in another. Deepen the outer corners and use a lighter shadow on the inner part of the eye. Then do the reverse. Brighten the area above and below the outer corner of your brow.

The two things that will dramatize the eye more than anything else are:
1. Blue eyeliner pencil applied on both upper and lower inner rim of eye.
2. Black mascara on curled lashes, well separated.

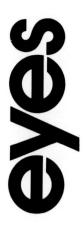

eyes

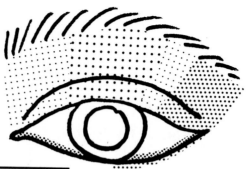

Almond or Oriental eyes

1. Apply a deep color (plum, light gray, navy, deep green) to the outer edge of the top lid. Ignore the natural crease. Build all color on outer third of eye.
2. Apply pastels (pink, yellow, ivory) to the inner corner of the eye. Carry up to brow and out.
3. Apply a shaft of bright reddish color or blusher directly above the iris, behind lashes, from the edge of the lid to the brow. Blend edges.
4. Apply a smudgy line under lower lashes. Continue it beyond outer corner of eye.
5. Line inside of eye, bottom rim only, with charcoal pencil.
6. Mascara on top and bottom lashes after curling. Brush upper lashes outward.

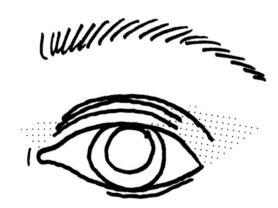

Crepey eyelids

1. Apply powder over the entire lid.
2. Then apply a touch of blusher on the outer corners of the eye.
3. Apply mascara on the outer corners of the top lashes only.
4. At all costs, avoid color. It will draw attention to the texture of your lids.

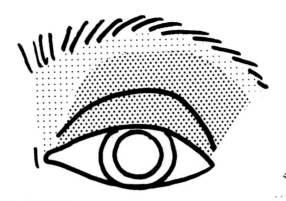

light bright medium dark

Bulging or puffy eyes

1. Powder entire eyelid from inner corner to brow and out to end.
2. Apply bright shadow (any reddish or yellow color will work) next to nose bone up into brow and across to the end, making an arch.
3. Put medium shadow (gray, blue, green, plum) on eyelid extending up behind crease. Make an arch. Blend dark and bright together well.
4. Do not use liner.
5. Apply mascara on top and bottom lashes —three times the amount on the bottom lashes.

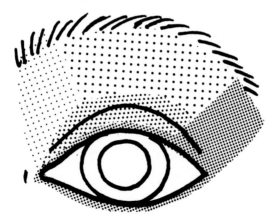

Perfect eyes

The perfect eye is large and lustrous. It has a generous lid and ample space between crease and brow. The lashes are thick and long. You cannot do anything wrong.
1. Powder and blend entire eyelid from inner corner up into brow and out.
2. Now experiment, using a combination of dark, light and bright colors. Be sure that all colors flow into each other—and remember that darkness causes the eye to recede and lightness to bring it forward.
3. Comb your lashes between layers of mascara or they will clump together.

14 EYE TRICKS

1. Always powder the entire eyelid, even if you don't plan to wear any eyeshadow. With-

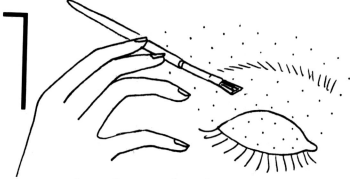

out eye makeup color, the powdered eye will at least give you some sort of a finished look. For shadow, you will be creating a matte surface to which the color will adhere smoothly. Any mistakes will also be more easily blended away.

2. For the best control, all powdered eyeshadow colors should be applied with a little brush and *not* with a sponge tipped applicator. Remember to blow away or tap excess powder off the brush; otherwise flecks will end up all over your cheeks.

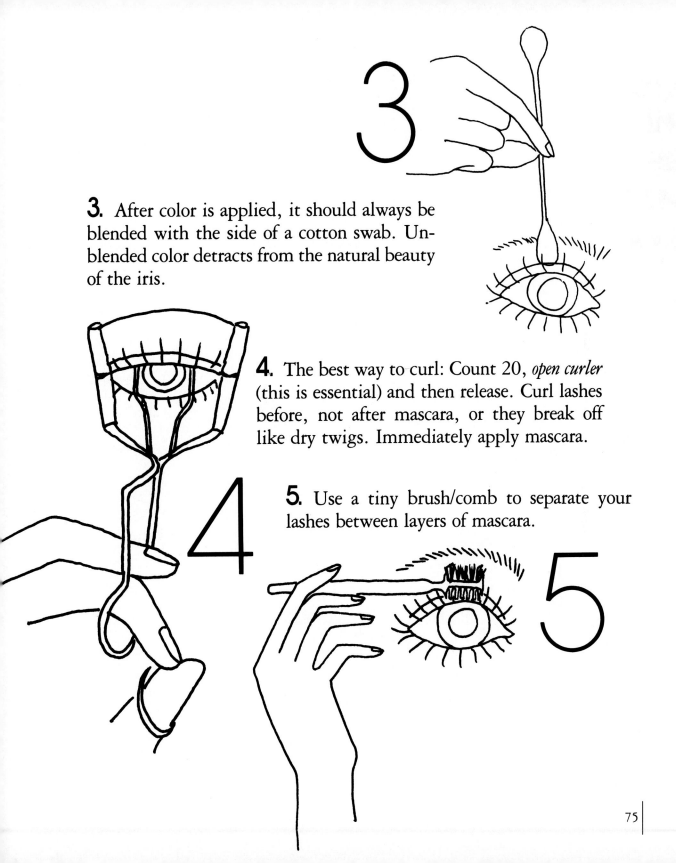

3. After color is applied, it should always be blended with the side of a cotton swab. Unblended color detracts from the natural beauty of the iris.

4. The best way to curl: Count 20, *open curler* (this is essential) and then release. Curl lashes before, not after mascara, or they break off like dry twigs. Immediately apply mascara.

5. Use a tiny brush/comb to separate your lashes between layers of mascara.

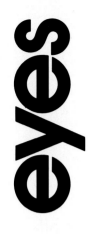

eyes

6. Dust lashes with loose powder between layers of mascara—this will thicken them.

7. Blue, black, charcoal or teal pencil lined on the inside rim of the eye makes the white appear whiter, the color of the iris deeper and the lashes thicker. (Find a soft "hypoallergenic" pencil so that it doesn't irritate you.)

8. If you use eyeshadow pencils for your lid color, be sure they are very soft, or they may damage the sensitive skin around the eye.

9. A good sharpener, to fit all sizes of pencil, is essential if the pencils are to do their work properly.

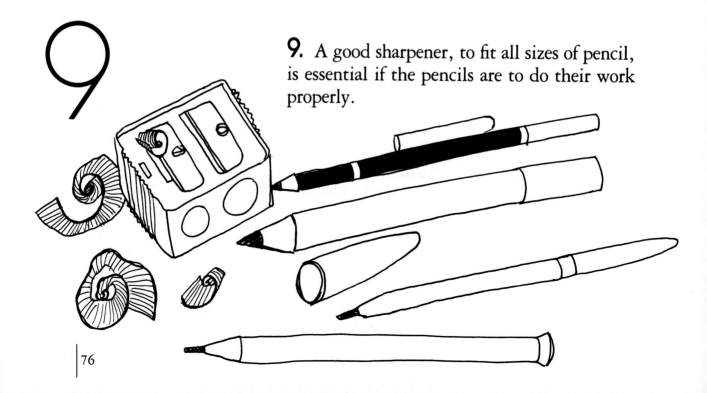

10. Liquid liners are treacherous for the non-professional; unless the liquid is half buffed away it will look hard and emphasize tiredness toward the end of the day.

11. Eye makeup must be removed *every* night. If you don't, the brittle mascara coated lashes will snap off as you turn on your pillow. The best way to remove mascara is to use eye makeup remover pads. Keep your eyes shut while you are stroking down gently over the eye area, and don't open them until you have rinsed with warm water on a clean washcloth. You can also use liquid eye makeup remover on a cotton ball in exactly the same way. Make sure it's nonirritating.

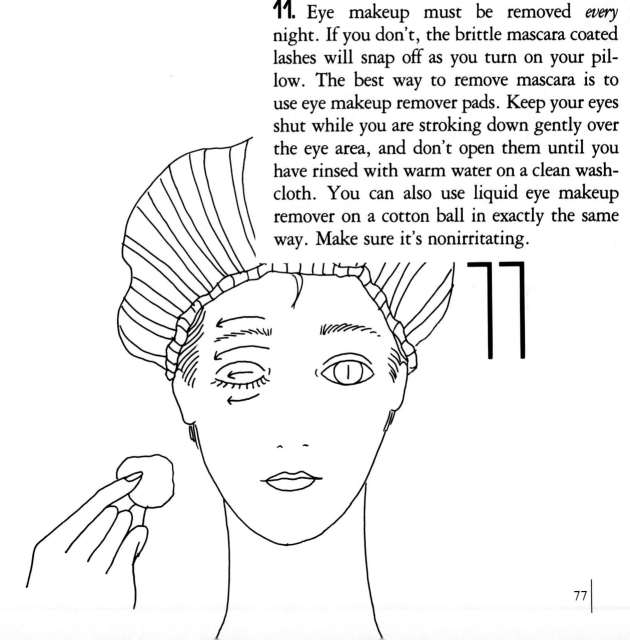

12. Don't wear mascara when you take an overnight plane flight. The dryness in the pressurized cabin will make your eyes sting.

13. Forget trying to match your clothes—use the color you're in the mood for. You can use a variety of shadows.

14. Remember that if you use too dark a shadow—or just one color—over the whole eyelid, the eye socket will appear to recede like a turtle withdrawing into its shell.

TIPS FOR CONTACT LENS WEARERS

1. It is much easier to apply eye makeup once your lenses are in.

2. Be sure to take out your lenses—soft or hard—before you remove your eye makeup. If you have extended wear lenses, use a hypoallergenic nonoily eye makeup liquid remover, on a gauze pad instead of on a cotton ball. Be especially careful *not* to open your eyes before rinsing with warm water on a clean washcloth.

MASCARA WISDOM

Twenty years ago, if you had asked one hundred women on the street which cosmetic product they wouldn't be caught dead without, ninety nine of them would have said "lipstick." Today it would be "mascara."

Ancient magic

It's all in the technique—mascara turns boring lashes into dynamite

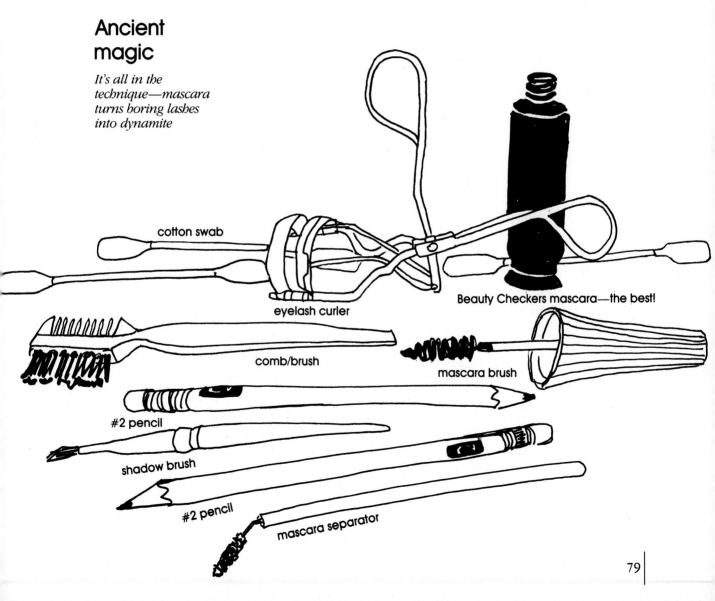

cotton swab

eyelash curler

Beauty Checkers mascara—the best!

comb/brush

mascara brush

#2 pencil

shadow brush

#2 pencil

mascara separator

eyes

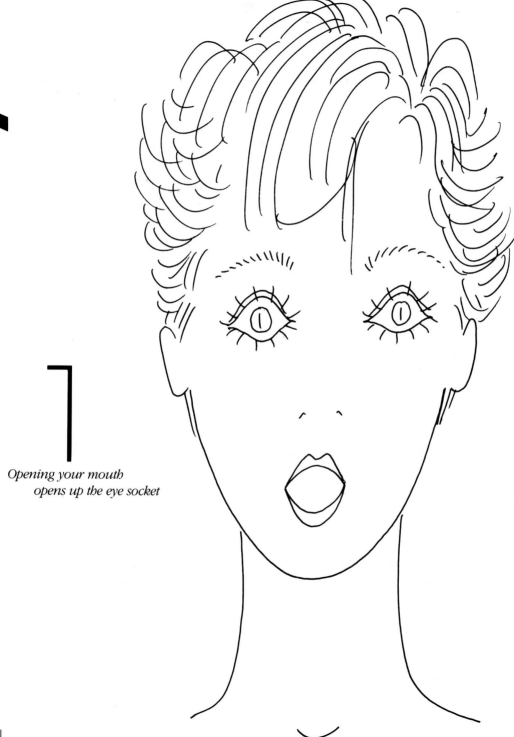

Opening your mouth
opens up the eye socket

This is because mascara does more—instantly—to glamorize you than anything else. The water soluble ones are easy to use and to remove. The "waterproof" mascaras cannot be "hypoallergenic"; the very ingredients that make them resistant to water may well cause irritation.

The correct way to apply mascara

1. Open your mouth. This will open up the eye socket, enlarging the area that you are working on.

2. (a) Top lashes: Start brushing at the midpoint of the eye, going straight up toward the brow. Now flick the outer lashes up and out, using the tip of the mascara wand to coat each individual lash. The inner corner is the trickiest, but don't ignore it, for it frames your eye. Here again, you will find that the tip of

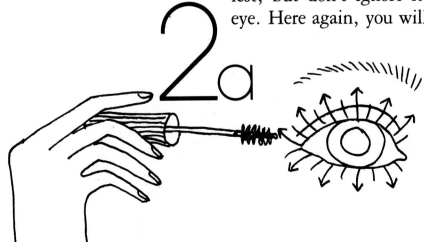

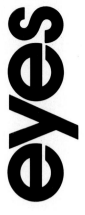

eyes

the brush works best. (b) Comb out the lashes before they dry, between layers, with a small brush/comb. If you hit skin anywhere along the line, stop *instantly* and with a moistened cotton swab, dab off the mistake.

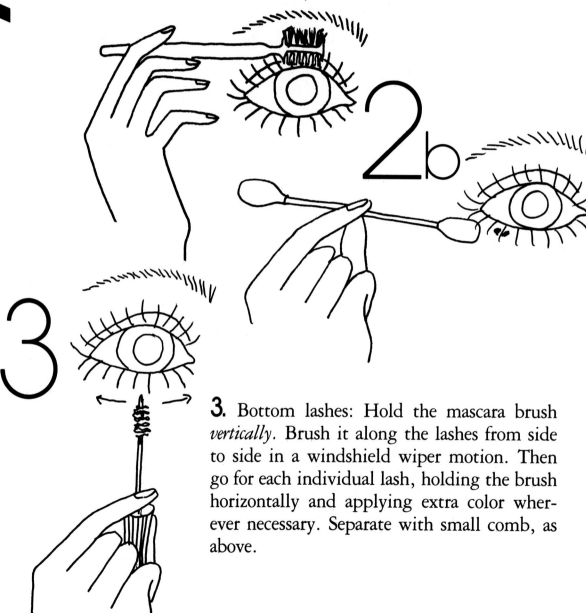

3. Bottom lashes: Hold the mascara brush *vertically*. Brush it along the lashes from side to side in a windshield wiper motion. Then go for each individual lash, holding the brush horizontally and applying extra color wherever necessary. Separate with small comb, as above.

4. Roll cotton swab dipped in loose powder under lower lashes to help prevent smudging.

Note: Everyone's lashes are stronger on one side than the other. The better ones are usually on the side you sleep on less. You'll need triple the quantity of mascara on the weaker side to compensate.

EYEBROWS— A JUNGLE

Women don't *see* their eyebrows—even when they are looking at them. Next time you go to a meeting or party, notice the eyebrows of the women around you. Most of them will be totally wrong.

The usual mistakes

• Women with naturally light brows will darken them.
• Brows that end in the right place are artificially extended downward.
• Natural cowlicks are ignored.

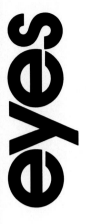

eyes

• Stray hairs are allowed to flourish and grow like the primeval jungle.

• Brows are plucked pencil thin to resemble the heroine of the late night movie.

Eyebrows should never distract from your eyes. Correct brows are rarely noticed because they are doing their job, drawing attention to the eyes themselves. It is when the brow is wrong that it is the first thing one sees. All the eye makeup expertise in the world will not help you if your brows do not have the proper shape and balance.

The overall stature and weight of your body will determine the size, thickness and color of your brows. If you are small-boned and delicate, of course your brows should be comparatively no less noticeable than if you were six feet tall.

Ways of improving your eyebrow
Shape

1. Put cold cream on your brows to soften and prepare them the night before you intend to pluck.

2. In the morning, remove any greasy residue left on your brows.

3. Always shape your eyebrows when you're standing up. This way you will work with

Put cold cream on your brows to soften and prepare them the night before you intend to pluck

the correct perspective. Peering down into a mirror will give you a distorted view and you'll pluck either too much or too little.

4. Now stand in a bright light (sunlight is best). Use a good magnifying mirror and a superb pair of tweezers. Always keep tweezers closed with a rubber band when not in use to protect the spring.

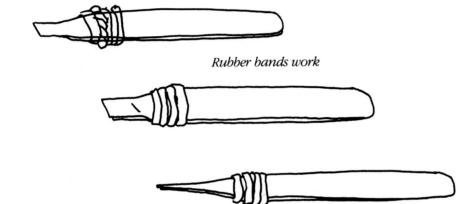

Rubber bands work

5. Your brow should start at a point directly above the inner corner of the eye, and the arch should be highest directly above the iris. The tail of the brow should extend just a touch beyond the outer corner of the eye—*never* pointing downward.

6. Pluck from underneath—one hair at a time. Pluck, stop, look and pluck again, until you get the right effect. Follow your natural browline; don't get carried away; and be sure to get a clean surface.

7. If your brows are sparse, fill in with a well-sharpened #2 writing pencil. Make tiny feather soft strokes, working in among existing eyebrow hairs. (You are coloring the underlying skin, not the hairs.) Brush upward briskly with an eyebrow brush or child's toothbrush.

8. If your brows are extra shaggy, unruly or full of cowlicks, you can do one of three things: You can either pluck them; trim them with small nail scissors (combing upward first to see just how much to trim); or take a tiny dab of false eyelash glue and stick them down.

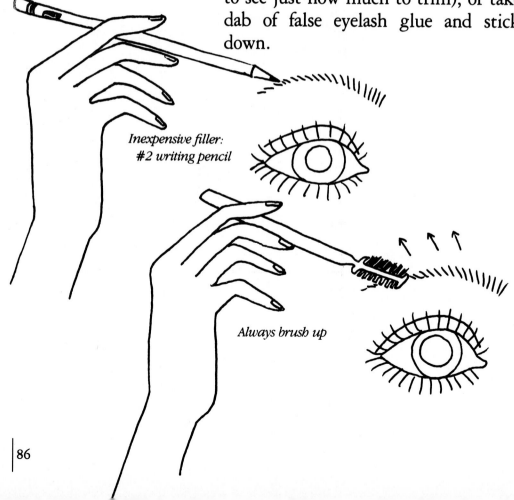

Inexpensive filler:
#2 writing pencil

Always brush up

Color

The color of your brows is just as important as the shape—and the color you were born with is seldom the one that does the most for you. Color is not sacred; changing it is usually a pleasant surprise. The correct color for most brows is about three shades lighter than your hair. Remember, nothing is as aging as thick, dark eyebrows. The older you are, the less brow you can carry.

There are some exceptions:

Blondes, redheads and white-haired women—all need brows three shades *darker* than their hair color.

If you live in an urban area, take advantage of the professional help available to you to correct and maintain your eyebrows. The ideal is to go to a professional every four to six weeks, keeping up the plucking between visits. Lightening the eyebrows is a tricky process which you should really not tackle yourself.

**The correct color
for most brows
is about three shades
lighter than
your hair**

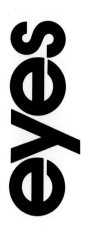

eyes

GLASSES— MEN *DO* MAKE PASSES AT GIRLS WHO WEAR THEM

Glasses don't have to work against you. Not only are they a wonderful prop, but many women actually look better in them. Make certain they fit securely without clamping your head or pinching the bridge of your nose. Also be sure that they don't keep sliding off. The tops of the frames should line up with your eyebrows; otherwise you will have two sets of parallel lines.

Choosing glasses should be easy. Here are some pointers:

The tops of your frames should line up with your eyebrows; otherwise you'll have two sets of parallel lines

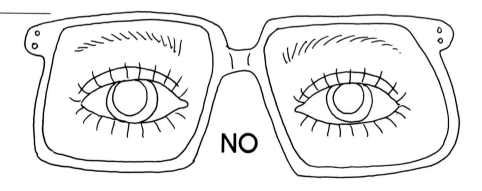

NO

1. Always stand in front of a full-length mirror when you are trying on frames—it's the only way to get a true picture of how they look on you.

2. There are no rules governing frame color —choose whatever makes you happy. However, various shades of tortoise shell are always safe. Glasses have become such a major investment that it will pay to be fairly conservative in your choice of color. You'll probably be looking at yourself through them for a long time.

3. Lenses tinted from dark to light are flattering even if the shading is very subtle.

4. Pink shaded lenses make your eyes look pink. If you don't mind looking like a rabbit, they're fine.

> Eye makeup needs
> to be intensified
> if you wear
> glasses

5. Eye makeup needs to be intensified if you wear glasses. Don't think that your unmadeup eyes will be hidden behind your everyday eye wear—they won't. They'll just look watery.

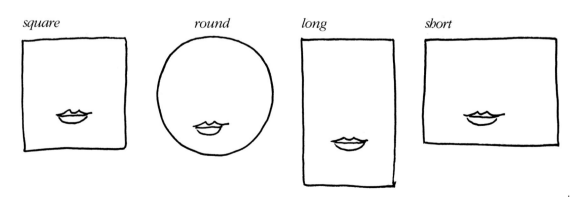

square *round* *long* *short*

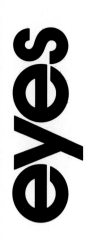

6. In general:

Square faces need large rounded or aviator-shaped frames.

Round faces need squarish or oblong frames.

Long faces need large, wide frames that cover much of the face.

Short faces are helped by rectangular or enormous round frames.

In other words, go in the opposite direction of your face shape, and thus balance it out.

round

short

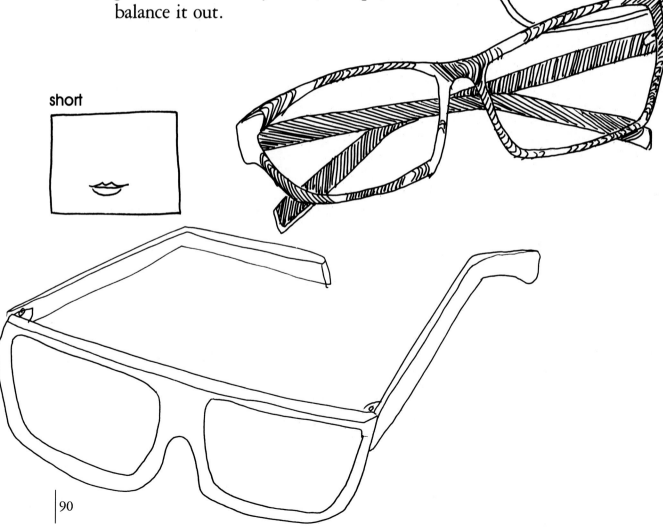

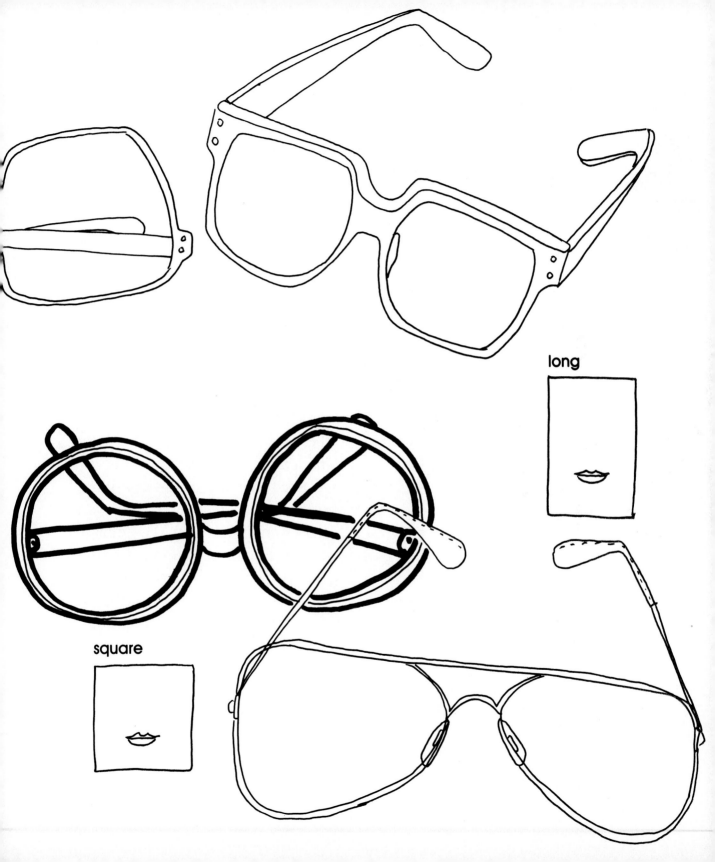

long

square

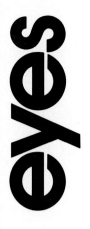

eyes

Sunglasses

Choose and try on your sunglasses in exactly the same way you do your regular ones. If you have a strong prescription the size of the glasses will be limited by it—if you do not, it can be a good idea to choose sunglasses on the large side for better sun protection. The shape you decide upon should be basically the same as your everyday pair.

Lens Color

Very dark glasses obscure the eyes; very light ones will not protect you from bright sunshine. Tinting the lenses from very dark to medium is the most effective and the most flattering. The color you choose should be soothing, but need not be dull—try gray, blue gray, pink gray or lavender rather than brown or green. Remember that the color of the glass will reflect onto your face. Tinting lenses is a process that can be reversed—be sure to get your optician to agree in advance to change the color of the lens if you don't like it. (There might be a slight additional charge.)

Everyone who wears glasses needs several pairs. You don't have to keep the same ones for ten years just because your prescription hasn't changed and the frame hasn't fallen apart. Explore the possibilities.

Thought it was easy?
How many did you
guess right?
The common denominator?
MASCARA

ANSWERS TO
EYE QUIZ

1		2	
3	4	5	6
7	8	9	10
11	12	13	
	14		

1. *Greta Garbo*
2. *Sophia Loren*
3. *Audrey Hepburn*
4. *Jacqueline Bisset*
5. *Elizabeth Taylor*
6. *Marilyn Monroe*
7. *Diahann Carroll*
8. *Barbra Streisand*
9. *Lee Remick*
10. *Joan Collins*
11. *Raquel Welch*
12. *Victoria Principal*
13. *Candice Bergen*
14. *Marlene Dietrich*

Our favorite is Garbo

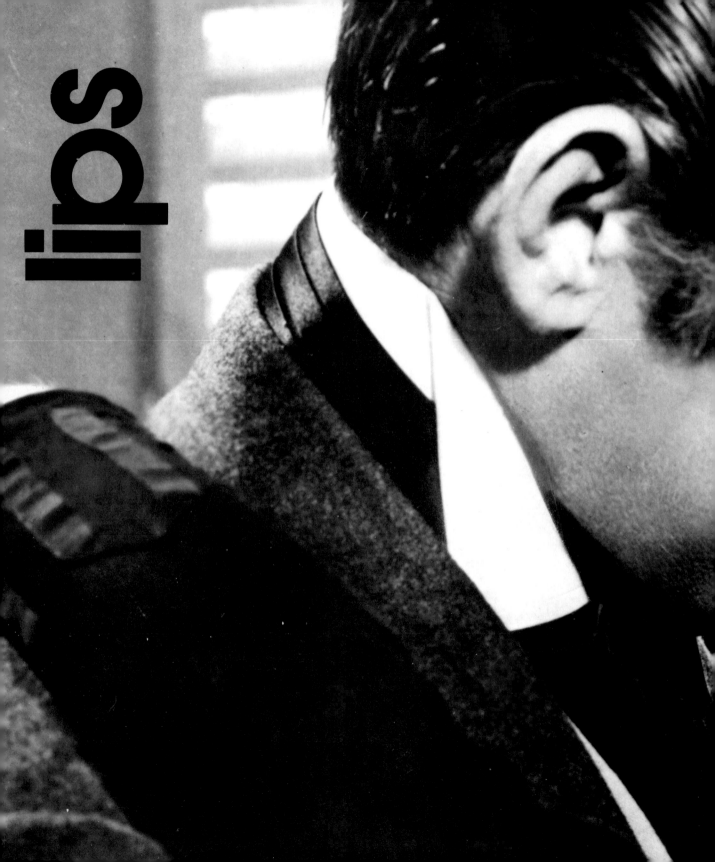

lips

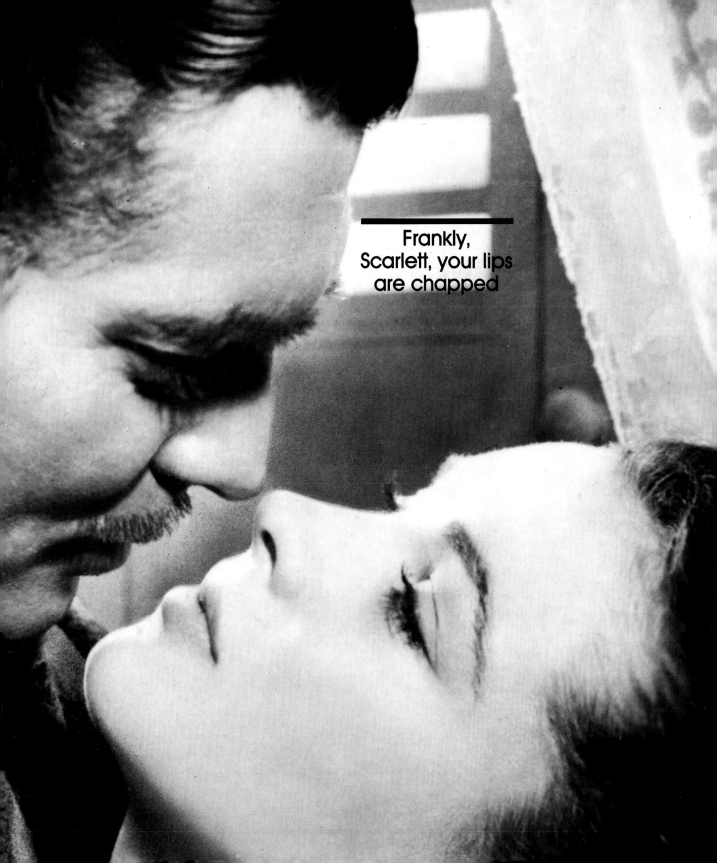

Frankly,
Scarlett, your lips
are chapped

lips

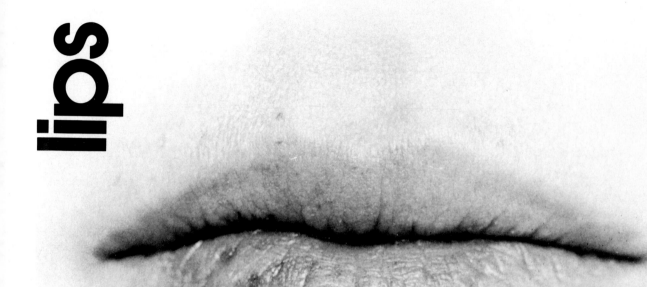

<u>Before</u>

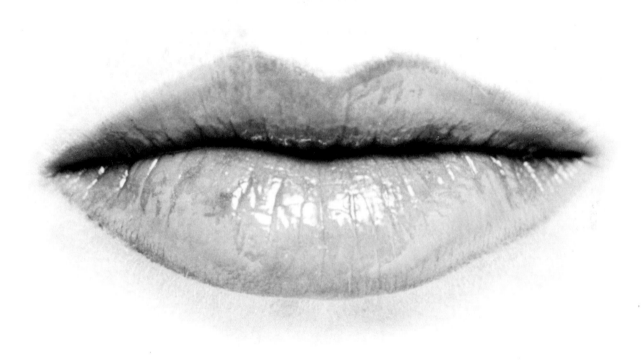

After

After the eyes, the lips contribute more than any other feature to the look of your face. Often women who dislike their lips think that by not using color they can get them to disappear. They are right—but what a waste. No lips are beyond redemption—whether it's a matter of texture, shape or color, there is a visual solution for everyone. Lips are inevitably sexy.

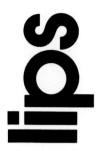

LIP PRODUCTS

PRODUCT	DRY LIPS	*(Instant disappearing act for all lip products)* OILY LIPS	NORMAL LIPS	MATURE LIPS
LIP FILLER	NO	**YES.** Another good step: Use makeup base or loose powder before anything else.	Sometimes	**YES**
LIP BALM *(Chap Stick, Blistex, "Boots": Every cosmetic line has one.)*	YES	NO	YES	**YES.** Center of lips only.
LIPSTICK (COLOR) *(with or without frost/translucent)*	**YES.** Ask for dry lip formula with moisturizers.	**YES.** Long lasting formula —if all else fails, food coloring as stain.	YES	**YES.** Long lasting formula
GLOSS *(clear or with color; in pot or plastic container with sponge applicator)*	**YES.** Over or instead of lipstick.	NO	**YES.** Over or instead of lipstick.	NO
LIP BRUSH *(for perfect outline and consistency)*	YES	YES	Preferably	YES
LIP LINER	NO	YES	If needed	NO

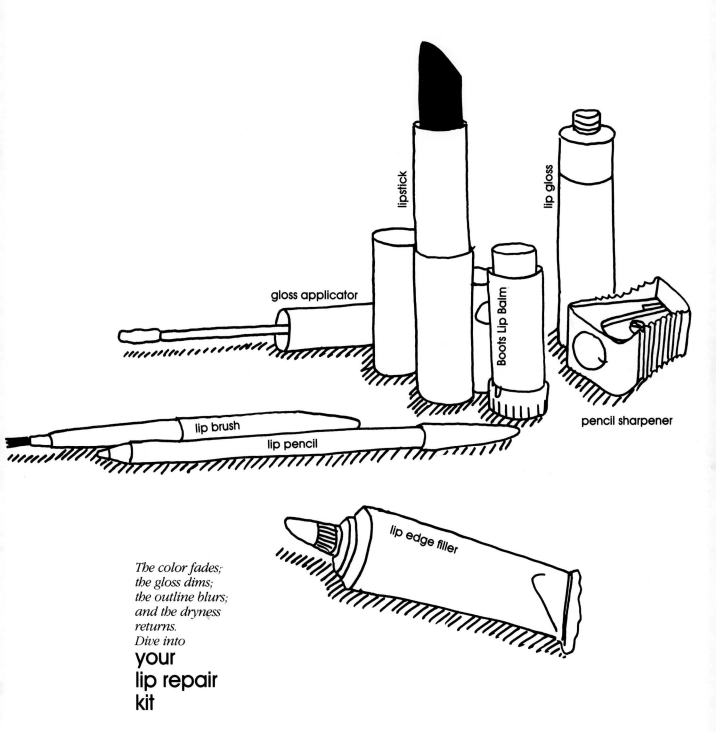

lipstick

lip gloss

gloss applicator

Boots Lip Balm

pencil sharpener

lip brush

lip pencil

lip edge filler

The color fades;
the gloss dims;
the outline blurs;
and the dryness
returns.
Dive into
your
lip repair
kit

lips

LIP POTENTIAL

When you look into the mirror, don't look only at your lips. Look at them as part of the whole face. This is the only way you can be objective.

Lips never match in size. For example, you think the top one is too thin; the bottom one too full. A question often asked at Beauty Checkers is: "What are perfect lips?" The answer: They do not exist. Lip fashions change with each generation. The day before yesterday's lips look dated.

TELLTALE TEXTURES

Believe it or not, tension has a lot to do with the texture of your lips; lip chewing and lip licking dry out the natural moisture. If you have one of these habits, you must constantly replenish the loss of moisture with a lip balm —about every half hour.

Scaly or parched lips are also caused by the following:

Sunburn: Prevent it by using a lip balm and a zinc oxide total sunblock.

Frost or extreme cold: Use a lip balm and apply it constantly. Avoid licking your lips.

Dry lips need constant moisture

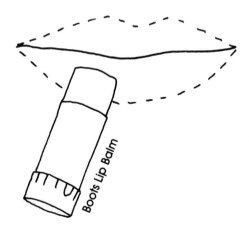

100

Sickness, medication, anesthesia: Vitamin E, taken internally (400 IUs—always check with your doctor first) and also applied externally in the form of a vitamin E stick.

Drugs, alcohol, smoking: All these are instantly ingested into the bloodstream, creating problems from within that affect your lips. Whatever balm you use will give only temporary relief. Tranquilizers and barbiturates can cause blisters around the mouth and flaking of the skin; cocaine and amphetamines or "uppers" make the lips and mouth very dry. People using even small quantities of these drugs constantly lick their lips, causing chapping and sores.

Allergy to lip products: Fragrances, dyes, waxes or iridescent qualities can cause allergies to lip products. If you know that you are allergic to fragrance, avoid buying strongly scented lipstick no matter how much you like the color. Lips are porous, just like the rest of your skin; dyes, waxes and iridescence are therefore absorbed (in miniscule quantities, true, but you can still be allergic to them). If your lips become sore or discolored, stop using everything for at least forty eight hours. Then apply lip balm or petroleum jelly, until they return to normal.

Sleeping with your mouth open: This could be the result of a medical or dental problem. Lip balm will help—temporarily.

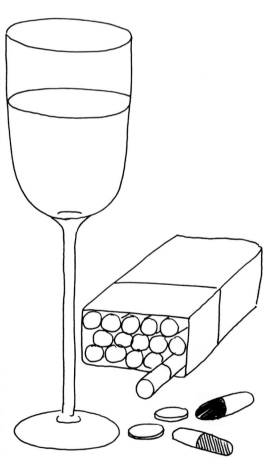

Lip negatives

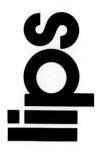

lips

Grainy, smudgy or freckled lips arrive suddenly, like your need for reading glasses. They're just something else to contend with.

Grainy lips: The surface of the lips, instead of being smooth and pliable, is crisscrossed by tiny wrinkles creating a leathery look.

Smudgy lips: The edges of the lips are characteristically uneven; they are punctuated by tiny vertical lines that run away with the lipstick you apply.

Here are our suggestions: For *grainy* or *smudgy* lips, *first,* use one of the new lip fillers only around the edges.

Lip filler is a white cream packed in a little tube. A drop is applied by finger and smoothed onto the lip edges before

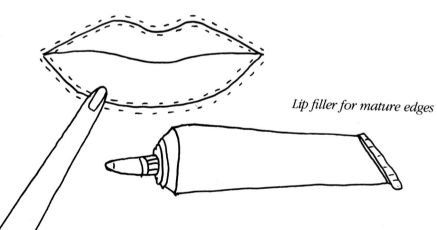

Lip filler for mature edges

any other lip product. It fills in the nooks and crannies and produces a smoothness that enables you to apply lip color evenly.

Second, use lip balm in the center of your lips. Or instead of balm, you can spread a little concealer around the edges of your lips, followed by powder directly on top of it. Warning: Dry lip time.

Then, go ahead and use lip color as usual. (Outlining with a lip pencil is helpful.)

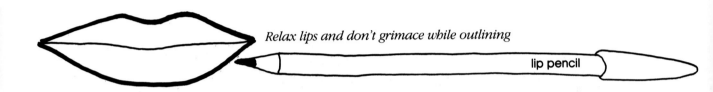

Relax lips and don't grimace while outlining

lip pencil

"Freckled" lips: The very things you may have observed on the backs of your hands (often caused by a lifetime of sun worship) can occur on the face—and yes, the lips.

For *freckled lips,* use a bright, distracting lip color—not a muddy one—and avoid lip gloss.

READING YOUR LIP COLOR

Really look at your lips, and reevaluate your lip color *daily*. It never stays the same.

Eighty percent of all women have blue lips—and the older you get, the bluer they get.

lips
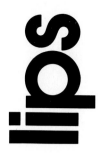

**Put your money
where your mouth is—
by the dozens**

---

newest favorite lipstick

✕ 12

Q. *What causes blue lips?*

A. Age, heredity, menstruation, tension, smoking, drugs, illness, medication, poor circulation, etc., and years of using a blue-based lipstick.

This blueness changes the lip color and you have to compensate by balancing it out. No lipstick will *ever* look exactly the same on you as it does in the tube, in the ads or on somebody else.

Colors change:
From orange to scarlet;
From pink to magenta;
From coral to deepest red;
From mulberry to oxblood;
From rust to brick;
From brown to MUD.

Learn how to produce the color that you want. For this you will need to experiment with mixing colors on a lipstick brush. Two colors and a gloss will nearly always give you a better color than just one lipstick. Try it—it's worthwhile, even if it is an extra step. (By the way, if you find a color you *love,* rush back and buy a dozen, and refrigerate them till you need them. It is an unwritten law that cosmetic companies discontinue colors that work for you.)

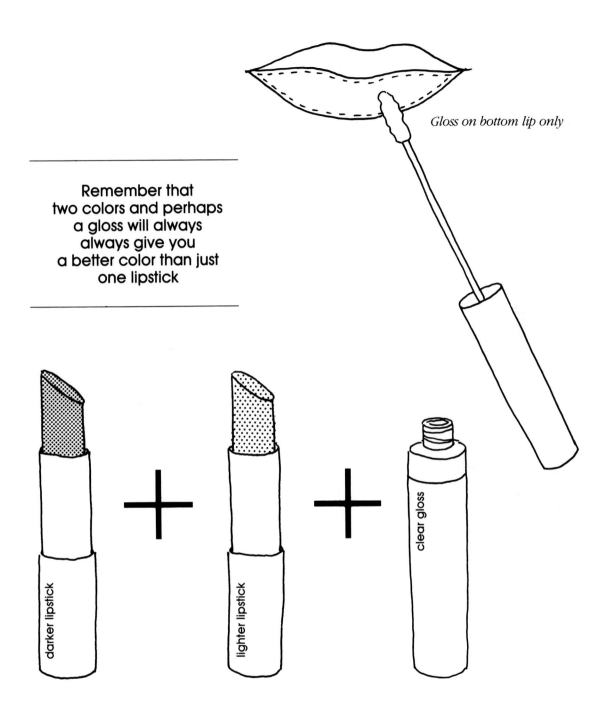

Gloss on bottom lip only

Remember that
two colors and perhaps
a gloss will always
always give you
a better color than just
one lipstick

darker lipstick

+

lighter lipstick

+

clear gloss

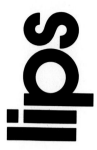
lips

Q. *How do I go about experimenting without buying dozens of wrong colors?*

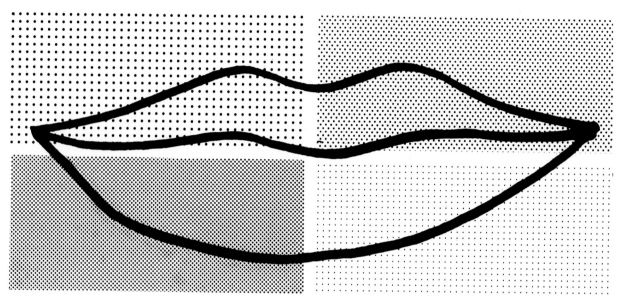

*Test four
different colors
on your lips—
not on the back
of your hand*

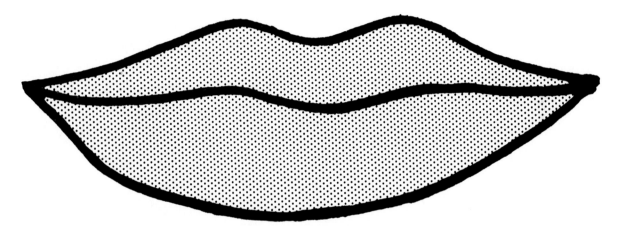

The right color makes it all work

**Always wipe off
the tester
with a clean tissue**

A. Go wherever the largest selection of testers is, usually a department store or large drugstore. (Always wipe off the tester with a clean tissue before using it.) Try a different color on each of the four quarters of your lips. Stand back, look at your face in the mirror: Focus on each individual color in succession. If you like one, gently wipe off the others, and try that color all over. If you don't like any of them, wipe them all off and repeat the process. (*Warning:* You can only do this experiment four times in one session—by then your lips will be discolored from all that wiping off, and no color will look right.)

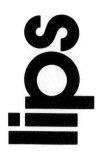

lips

Q. *Do I change my lip color to match what I'm wearing?*

A. No, never. Whatever color makes you look pretty is correct.

Q. *Do I change my lip color according to the time of day?*

A. Yes, and here is a guide:

Early AM exercises: Lip balm only.

Morning: Melon, pink, coral; the key word is "soft."

Noon: As above, plus gloss.

Evening: Time for drama: bright reds, rich magentas, deep burgundies, plus gloss.

Other situations: Sports, snow, sea, gardening, country mornings—we don't believe in lip color for the above. Protect your lips with a balm; if you feel you must have color, a very light gloss.

LIP TIPS

1. Lip-liner pencil: It has to be sharp. Blunt tip = fuzzy outline.

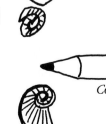

Constants

2. Lip liner must be unobtrusive; it should not make the lips two tone. Apply before lipstick, and smudge into the lips with your pinky. Follow your natural lip line, or create one to enlarge or shrink your mouth, as needed.

3. Lipstick should be applied with a lip brush. It may be awkward at first but stick with it and you will find that it becomes second nature. The brush gives special control—and can also be used to outline the mouth if using a lip pencil doesn't work for you.

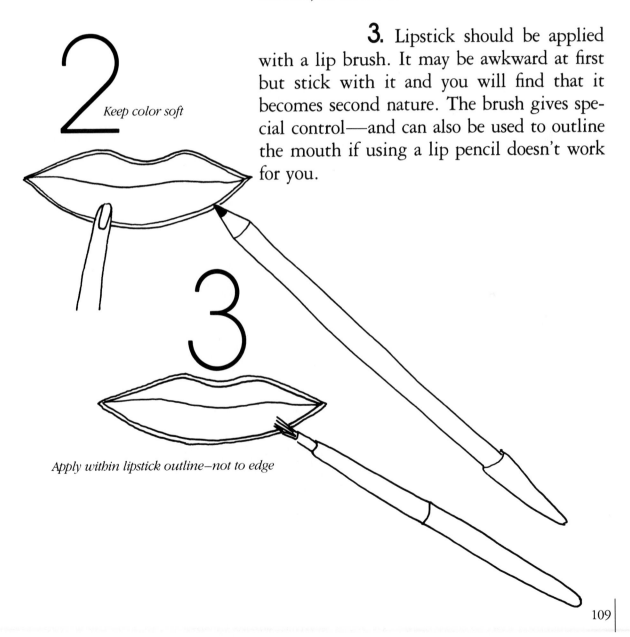

Keep color soft

Apply within lipstick outline–not to edge

LIP TRICKS

lips

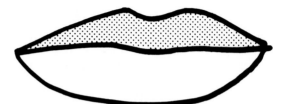

1. Thin top lip.
Light lipstick on top will balance out size.
No color on bottom lip.

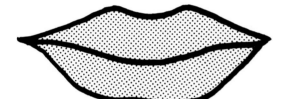

2. Undefined edge.
Outline lips with a melon pencil. Fill in with
lighter shade.

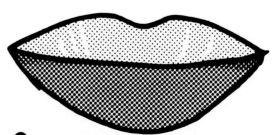

3. Full bottom lip.
Darker lipstick shade on bottom lip. Gloss
over lighter shade on top lip.

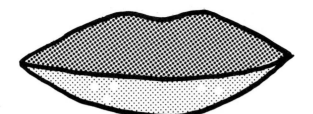

4. Full upper lip.
Darken top lip with deeper lip shade. Gloss over
lighter shade on bottom lip.

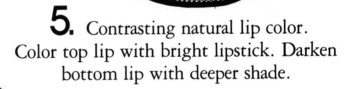

5. Contrasting natural lip color.
Color top lip with bright lipstick. Darken
bottom lip with deeper shade.

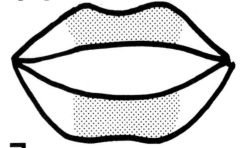

6. Contrasting natural lip color—reversed.
Brighten bottom lip. Darken top lip.

7. Smudgy lips.
Use concealer over entire edge of both lips.
Use pinkish lipstick color in center of mouth only,
avoiding edges.

lips

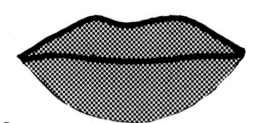

8. Undefined edge to top lip.
Outline top lip to provide definition. Fill in
both lips with lipstick.

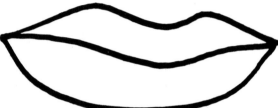

9. Wavy, uneven color.
Apply lip moisturizer and foundation, then
clear gloss all over both lips.
No lipstick color.

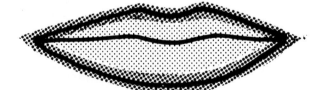

10. Thin lips.
Redefine lips by blotting out outside edges with
foundation and powder. Redraw mouth
just outside natural lip line with lip brush or pencil.
Fill in with favorite color lipstick.

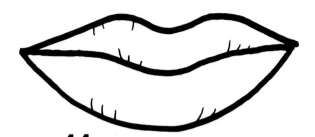

11. Chapped lips.

Apply lip balm constantly, even before sleep. Avoid all lip color until healed.

---

12. Perfect lips.

Lucky you—anything goes!

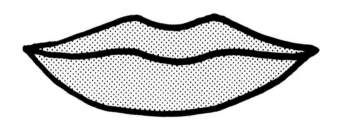

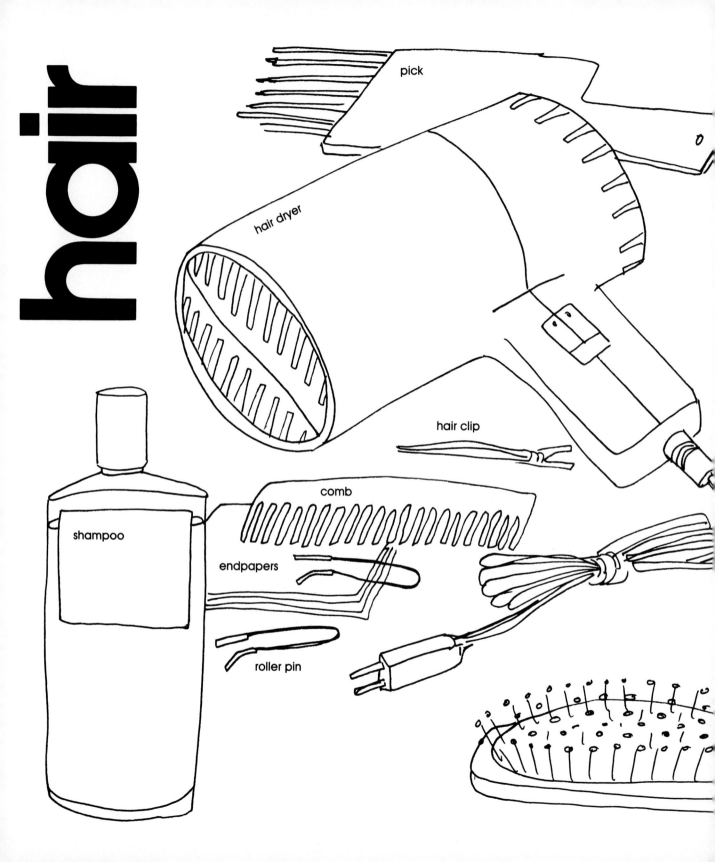

hair

pick

hair dryer

hair clip

comb

shampoo

endpapers

roller pin

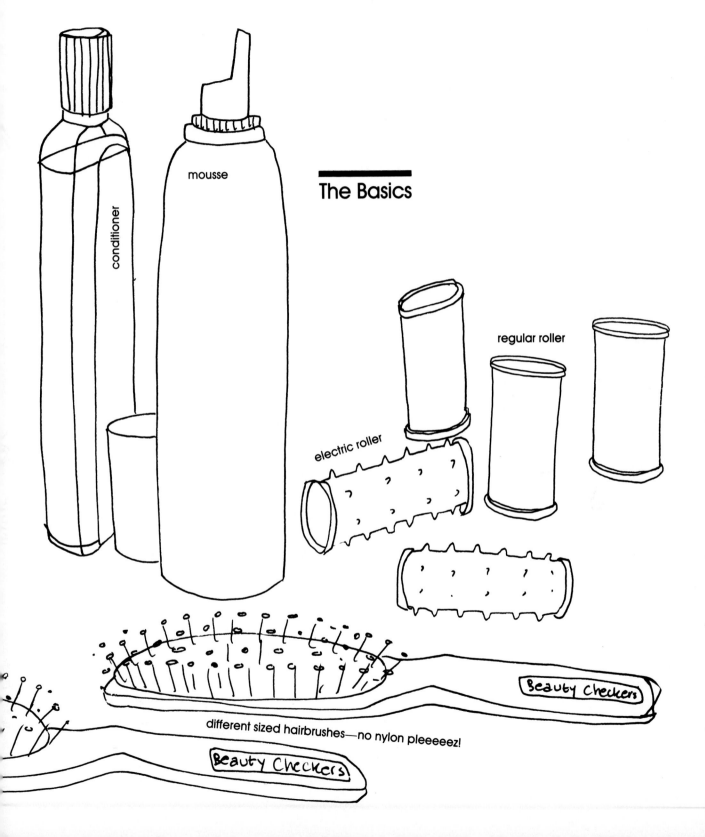

conditioner

mousse

The Basics

electric roller

regular roller

Beauty Checkers

different sized hairbrushes—no nylon pleeeeez!

Beauty Checkers

hair hair hair hair

Hair is not a thing unto itself—it is part of a total image. To put hair into its proper perspective, look at yourself in a full length mirror wearing your normal makeup. Try on, in succession, several different kinds of clothing: jeans and sweaters, a business outfit, then something dressy. Does your hair contribute to each effect? Study yourself every which way. Be ruthless: Does your hair look good from the front? From the back? In profile? If everything works *except* your hair, it's time to do something about it.

TROUBLE AT THE TOP

Is it the length? The style?
A lack of vitality?
Is it lank? Or dull?
Overprocessed?
Overconditioned?
Do you look like Ms. Mouse?
Do you have dead, split ends?
Is it unmanageable?
Does it look like the work
of loving hands at home?
Is it boring?

Any of the above can easily be taken care of on a Tuesday morning. (The best hairdresser in town is usually closed on Monday.)

No matter how you feel, the

sight of a wonderful healthy mane in the mirror has to make you happier. Getting your hair to look good every morning is what launches your day. Good health is the basis of good hair—but to keep it healthy requires constant effort. It is essential to have a daily maintenance regime, just as you have for your face. Trillions of dollars are spent annually on developing hair products, so that anything you need is available in any price range. Alas, trial and error is the only way to discover what's right for you—even with the help of an expert. Once you find what works, stick with it.

The following is the ideal routine. Being realists, we know that it can't fit into everyone's lifestyle, but, with slight variations, it can become your very own discipline.

DAILY REGIMEN

Wash your hair every day.

Do not attack the scalp. Massage it gently.

Commercial shampoos are all too strong. Dilute the shampoo—about one part shampoo to three parts water—in an empty plastic bottle, and shake.

Rinse, rinse, rinse! You can never rinse too much. If you take three minutes to wash, you need six minutes to rinse

If you take
three minutes to wash,
you need six minutes
to rinse for
squeaky clean hair

Eat foods rich in
vitamins and proteins
for shiny,
healthy hair

for squeaky clean hair. Those tiny white flakes that look like dandruff may only be shampoo residue from insufficiently rinsed hair.

As for conditioning, you may need to condition your hair daily, weekly or not at all; it depends on the texture of your hair and whether it is chemically treated in any way (streaked, colored, permed or straightened). Treated hair must be conditioned each time it is washed.

Scalp conditioning is different from hair conditioning. Your scalp may be oily and the ends of your hair dry, or the reverse. Consult your hairdresser for the right scalp conditioner to use, and the frequency with which to use it.

Don't yank at your hair or try to comb through wet hair in one fell swoop. Deal with tangles by gently combing out each section.

If you blow dry, avoid pulling and don't overdry.

Do take vitamins (Bs and Es) and eat foods rich in protein for shiny, healthy hair. Know that neither vitamins nor protein applied *externally* will do anything to help your hair . . . no matter what the label says.

THE ROOT OF HAIR PROBLEMS

Many women have hair problems. Often they

are caused by chemical abuse of the hair: Perming, bleaching, straightening, coloring, etc. However skillfully these procedures are carried out, and however mild the products used, they will eventually harm the hair. Obviously, we don't expect you to abandon these practices altogether any more than we propose jettisoning your mascara. The hair, like the face, needs constant work to keep us looking good; but we must at least learn to compensate for the inevitable damage done. This is why the daily maintenance regime is of such great importance.

Hair fallout

Women go into shock when they see strands of their hair lying on the pillow—or lining the tub. Yet this is the most common hair problem and it has a variety of causes.

1. **Heredity:** The tendency to lose your hair can be hereditary—but just because you have a predisposition to hair loss doesn't necessarily mean that it will actually happen.

2. **Stress:** There is a proven medical connection between hair loss and stress. Stress promotes a certain chemical reaction in the hair, and if the hair follicle is genetically sensitive, the hair may fall out. Get rid of the stress and the hair will usually grow back.

3. **Physical trauma:** Pulling or tugging at

Get rid of
the stress and hair will
usually grow back

A constant lifetime
maintenance program
should
retard the
thinning process

the hair; tight braids, ponytails and chignons; straightening; tight rollers (does anyone still use them?); fast blow drying; intense heat drying; teasing; back combing; heavy spraying; as well as the aforementioned overprocessing—all contribute to hair loss.

4. Pregnancy: During pregnancy the hair is usually thick and plentiful, but between the sixth and seventh month after delivery, hair will often fall out. This is only temporary— it will grow back as the hormonal balance of the body returns to normal. After your first pregnancy, however, it will never be exactly as it was before.

5. Illness: Hair may fall out as a result of high fever, anemia, thyroid or ovarian problems; sometimes this hair loss may be the first indication that something is wrong.

6. Anesthesia and medication: These sometimes cause hair loss, though the hair should grow back.

7. Age: Older hair is unavoidably thinner, but a constant lifetime maintenance program should retard the thinning process.

Parenthetically, some experts believe that there are definite times of the year (spring and fall) when we "molt," just like birds. Remember, too, that most hair fallout in women is reversible.

Hair, like skin, is a natural survivor—invest in it and it will reward you.

The beauty profession has developed its own group of specialists, problem solvers who abound in most urban centers. Their knowledge is expensive—but infinitely worthwhile. We have interviewed a number of these specialists and want to share their wisdom with you.

THE CUT

Like your makeup, your hairstyle must be adapted to the different stages in your life. The hair of a woman in her forties differs from that of a woman in her twenties. For many women, long hair is a symbol—of glamour, youth and femininity. Tresses are hung on to for a number of other reasons: It's easy to make a ponytail (which is where most long hair winds up); it's economical, requiring very little investment in haircuts; it's simple, requiring less shampooing. Let's deal with the effects of these practices one by one:

• Ponytails cause tremendous stress on the hair and result in prematurely receding hairlines.

• If hair is not trimmed every six to eight weeks, you'll get split ends which will run up the hair shaft like runs in pantyhose.

• Shampoo at least every other day or your hair will be dull and lifeless.

• Older men may love long

hair hair hair

hair, but younger ones definitely feel short hair is sexier.

Long hair was the 1960s, the era when the ultimate was to have a great mane of shiny, "swinging hair." Today, a good hairdresser will show a client how to work with her individual hair texture—there are endless options. It doesn't have to be long to look its best.

The time to cut long hair comes when you know it isn't helping your face. There is nothing more disconcerting than seeing a long haired woman walking down the street and realizing as you pass her that she's twenty from the back and sixty from the front. If this hits a nerve, get thee to a hairdresser! Don't wait for an emotional trauma to send you fleeing in search of transformation. Do it while you are feeling good about yourself and receptive to change. If the cut you get isn't quite what you had imagined, it's certainly no cause for alarm. After all, it's only hair, and it will grow back.

Texture

All of our experts say that the most difficult textures to work with are the two extremes: very fine, sparse hair and dense, thick hair. (Hair that has been straightened is also a problem because it has none of its own wave pattern to follow in a haircut.) Thick, frizzy hair will look terrific and become infinitely

> Shampoo at least every other day or your hair will be dull and lifeless

> The time to cut long hair comes when you know it isn't helping your face

easier to manage if kept really short. Baby-fine hair, which should be no more than chin length, desperately needs a perm, to give it body, or to be colored, which adds body of its own. Between these two extremes are all other hair textures, which are far more versatile. But, before you do anything about your hair, you must find out what your hair texture really is.

Particular hairdressers specialize in specific hair textures, and when you are making your appointment, be sure to ask for a (free) consultation before your actual haircut date. Go in with your hair at its worst, and then talk it out with the hairdresser of your choice. If you don't like what you hear, or you get uncomfortable vibes, don't go back (but do cancel the appointment, of course). It is *very* important to have a good understanding with the person who is going to be doing the work—and all hairdressers welcome this five minutes of discussion; it makes their job much easier in the end. Hairdressers do better work on a secure client.

Now you've had your haircut and your hair is in marvelous shape. Discuss its upkeep with the expert. Long hair needs cutting every four to six weeks. With short hair, there is no hiding, so it must be cut every three to four weeks. A good professional perm/body wave helps you hide a bad haircut or growing-out hair, by making maintenance

Thick, frizzy hair will look terrific and become infinitely easier to manage if kept really short

easier and adding volume to the hair. If your hair is short, the wave is constantly being trimmed away, so you'll need three to five perms in the course of a year. Longer hair can go as much as six months.

Metamorphosis

Changing your hairstyle, like changing your clothes or your makeup, should not be traumatic. On the contrary, it is something to look forward to. Once you have worked it out with your hairdresser, relax and enjoy it. If you do decide to bring in a picture, it is a good starting point, but treat it only as a suggestion. No two heads of hair ever look exactly alike. What you see in the picture has to be adapted to you.

Most beauty books give you face shapes and the "right" corresponding hairstyles. We feel that this approach is misguided. Today it is the hair texture, the lifestyle and the age of a woman, not her face shape, that determines the way she should wear her hair. A sensitive hairdresser will first listen to what you have to say, and then study you feature by feature, using your hair as a complement. Hairdressers love to perform a total transformation. However, a one step change from long hair to short hair may be a mistake. Newly cut hair needs time to reshape itself—it is therefore best for it to be cut in two stages, the second after a week or

Long hair needs cutting every four to six weeks

two and several shampoos.

Finally, hair should not overwhelm or distract from a good face. Conversely, a more involved hairdo will enhance a less attractive one.

CASTING THE DYE

Newly cut hair needs time to reshape itself

There are few of us bold enough to pick up scissors and cut our own hair; and yet we do not hesitate to improvise with home hair-color kits. Our color experts agree that women are very naive when it comes to hair color.

There is nothing wrong with home color products; after all, they are basically the same ones that professionals use—but *they* read the instructions and follow them to the letter. Coloring instructions are not like cooking recipes, where a pinch of this and a touch of that may be a smashing success. Don't be creative. Just do exactly what you are told. Otherwise, blame only yourself and not the manufacturer.

Don't forget that hair is constantly growing and oxydizing, and the color you apply simply will not stay the same. If you repeat the rinse before the period of time specified in the instructions, you will eventually get *color build up*—and then it will be

Don't be creative—
just do exactly
what you are told

time for expensive professional hair color correction.

A bad color job is a more serious problem than a bad haircut, because it cannot be hidden. It takes an awful lot of time, effort and money to reverse the damage.

The basics:
when, why and how

Blond hair has long been a fantasy, with each age having its idols. Today they are Princess Di, Christie Brinkley, Cheryl Tiegs and Linda Evans; Marilyn Monroe, Jean Harlow and Veronica Lake are part of our hair-itage.

We used to start coloring our hair when it turned gray. Today we also do it simply for a change, and we start much earlier —often in high school.

The paler the shade, the better it sells—instant glamour is within everyone's grasp. However, we should realize that the reality will never match the picture on the package. The shade you get will be a blend of your own color and the color from the bottle. So don't be disappointed.

Black is the second best seller —followed by various shades of *brown*. *Red* accounts for only ten percent of the market. Red is understood and bought in the larger urban areas, but most reject it as being too extreme, and tend to consider it "brassy."

126

Streaks, highlights, glazes and all over hair color

The shade you get
will be a blend
of your own color
and the color from the
bottle

The great advantage of
highlighting
is that the roots
don't show up as quickly

Streaks, highlights and glazes are the closest thing to sunstreaked hair. They differ from all over hair color in that they are usually done around the hairline and the front of the head, without touching the actual roots or scalp. Since the overall color of the hair is not being changed, one can say that it looks more natural, which is what most women want. The great advantage of highlighting is that the roots don't show up as quickly.

One of our experts says that she streaks forty five percent of her clientele, while fifty five percent get a single process. Another tells us that she only does streaking because it achieves the right effect without being unnecessarily drastic. A third expert does mostly highlighting and glazing. He finds that his clients frequently want to change their hair color (a new concept for American women). Since the glazes quickly oxidize and wash out, they allow for new color within a matter of weeks.

Another colorist streaks approximately fifty percent of her clients, while the rest get "single process color." This differs from streaking in that the color is applied to the scalp and covers the roots as well as the shaft. It is ideal for gray haired women who

> The closer you stick to your own natural hair color, the less frequent the touch ups

really don't want their gray to show. With "two process color," the hair is first bleached, and then another color is applied to the bleached hair. This is very destructive and involves monthly attention because the roots grow out.

Once you start coloring your hair, you are committed and you must constantly work at keeping it up. Of course, the closer you stick to your natural hair color, the less frequent the touch ups. Older women with all over gray should not try to duplicate their original color if it was dark—the result will be aging and unflattering. It is *always* advisable to go a few shades lighter.

Based on our personal experience, and our research with hair experts, we are more convinced than ever that perms and colors do not mix. It's just too much for the hair. If you want to throw caution to the wind, however, and you happen to have dead, straight, mousy hair, at least wait a month after having it permed, and then color it. If your hair is simply frosted, and you perm it, you will be dealing with two kinds of hair: bleached and normal. The bleached hair will frizz; the normal hair will not respond. In other words, as with bleached hair, the perm will not work at all.

TRAVELING WITH YOUR HAIR

A successful lifestyle today often means being on the move. And as we crisscross the globe, our hair has to look just as terrific as it does at home. This means that we have to carry a mini beauty salon with us. It should consist of whatever you generally use to do your hair at home: Shampoo, conditioner, blow dryer, electric rollers, endpapers, hair clips and, believe it or not, a net to keep the whole thing together at night. Trips to particular climates demand special products: A woman on a skiing trip needs mousse for hair control and a wooden comb to balance out static electricity. In a tropical climate, she needs baby oil to comb through her hair for protection against sun and salt water.

Remember that if you have a good basic haircut, doing your own hair will be infinitely more to your liking than the work of an unfamiliar hairdresser whom you may never see again. If you normally get a weekly or biweekly shampoo and set, however, by all means go to the local hairdresser, but take along your own shampoo, conditioner and rollers. If your trip is an extended one and your hair is colored, take with you not only your written formula, but also its separate ingredients.

Take along your
own shampoo, condi-
tioner and rollers

The ideal
travel companion is a
head of wash and
wear hair

In some areas,
the hair never gets to
feel clean, and you may
have to consider buying
bottled water for the
final rinse

Obviously, the ideal travel companion is a head of wash and wear hair—and if you are going on a long trip, you might consider experimenting with a no fuss hairstyle. Then again, if you are traveling abroad and decide to take a friend's recommendation on the best salon in town, you should treat the visit as part of the pleasure of the trip. Of course, you may not emerge looking familiar, but this is part of the excitement.

It needn't be Perrier, but . . .

Water varies from place to place and you have to make adjustments for it. Shampoo clings to hair that is washed in hard water, so you have to triple your rinse time. In some areas, the hair never gets to feel clean and you may have to consider buying bottled water to wash it in—as Elizabeth Taylor did when she was filming *The Bluebird* in Leningrad.

Water pressure is another variable, and it will influence the length of the whole cleansing process.

HAIR POLLUTION

The country dweller will find that in the city —any city—pollution settles instantly in the hair, which means that it has to be washed twice as often. Heat and humidity (great for thin hair) will frizz normal hair into an intractable mass. Dry air makes curly hair straight, and straight hair limp. Dampness curls. Cold weather means head hugging hats, which lead in turn to flattening, static electricity and increased oiliness of the scalp —no matter what type of hair you have. Finally, remember that the cabin pressure in an airplane affects everyone's hair—adversely.

> **Dry air makes curly hair straight, and straight hair limp. Dampness curls**

The burn

The sun will dry, oxidize and change the color of all hair. If your hair is colored, the sun will obliterate subtleties and produce a cotton candy effect; and wearing a straw hat to protect it from the sun may not help, as the concentrated heat is just as harmful.

To prevent sun and salt water from damaging your hair, you should saturate it with either baby oil, conditioner or suntan lotion before sunning yourself. If you swim in a pool, be sure to wear a well fitted swimming cap, or the oil from your head will interfere with the pool's filtering system. It's for your own sake, too: Chlorine can turn colored hair green.

Chlorine can turn
bleached hair green

Just as you shouldn't
use detergent soap
on your face,
you shouldn't use a
detergent
shampoo

POTIONS AND LOTIONS

There are far too many hair products on the market. The first thing to remember, as with cosmetics, is that more expensive doesn't necessarily mean better. All hair products contain basically the same ingredients. Just as you shouldn't use a detergent soap on your face, avoid a detergent shampoo. Remember that all those magic ingredients that make the prices soar are just so many words.

Shampoos

As in cosmetics, there are no hard and fast rules. A dollar shampoo may do wonders for Mary and make Sally's hair fall out. It's a matter of susceptibility. The shampoo has to suit *your hair,* and as we've said earlier in this chapter, once you've found what works for you, stick to it.

In the world of beauty, the "natural" product does not exist. What is "natural" anyway? Even we are not "natural" —we are composed of chemicals. We eat, sleep and breathe by a series of chemical processes. If a "natural" cosmetic product is to have a shelf life, it has to contain some preservatives. Without them, the product would be rancid in a week. "Natural" products won't hurt you, but they are no better than those which don't claim to be "natural."

Conditioners

Conditioners work beautifully in hair that has been chemically processed. Tangled hair also needs a conditioner after shampooing to make it easy to comb through, though some people cannot use conditioners at all—it takes all the life and body out of their hair. In any case, use the minimum, and don't condition the area near the hair root, where the oil glands are, or you'll wind up with greasy hair. The ends need the conditioning. Choose your conditioner by the same rules as your shampoo —trial and error.

In the world of beauty, the word "natural" doesn't exist

Mousse

Mousse is the new kid on the block. It is used to control and shape the hair in much the same way as setting lotion or hair spray. It is especially effective in the summer, and for involved hairstyles. If you have short hair that needs a cut every three weeks, mousse can be used to shape it and extend the life of the cut. Its only drawback: It attracts every impurity floating in the air—which means daily shampooing is essential.

Other hair products will be discussed in the glossary at the end of the book.

Choose your conditioner by the same rules as your shampoo— trial and error

hair hair hair hair

Hair independence

In the 1970s, hairdressers began to ask their clients about the way they lived before they began cutting. The daily life of the contemporary woman had simply become too complicated for her to remain a slave to her hair. Today hair independence is the norm. When professional help is needed, we go to the experts. For the daily routine, we rely on ourselves.

The reckoning

A hairdresser's bill can sometimes put us into a state of shock. This is perhaps because we haven't allowed for the fact that we must pay for everything that is done to us in a beauty salon. Few of us have the courage to turn down a conditioner when the shampooer whispers that we need it. Suggestions like this are all made very casually, and are not intended to be misleading. Each item does add up, however.

One way of eliminating a step is to come in with freshly shampooed hair. Another is to go without a blow dry after the cut. Even if you sit under a heat lamp, you pay for it!

The gratuity

Women are often in a quandary about how

> Today,
> hair independence
> is the norm

> We must
> pay for everything
> that is
> done to us in a
> beauty salon

much to tip, how to tip and when to tip. Tipping is an expression of our appreciation for services rendered. Tipping also takes into consideration the actual time the operator has spent with us.

Owners of smaller salons accept tips, as do their staffs. The superstars who charge a premium for their services usually refuse tips.

This is simply to give you a point of reference. It is always a good idea to ask at the desk what the normal tipping rates are—though needless to say, no one will check on what you give.

Some salons expect more of you than others, but ultimately the tip is what *you* consider fair. Don't be anxious about it. You will get the optimum services which will be quite unrelated to the amount you decide to leave. Remember, the purpose of tipping is to reflect the degree of *your* satisfaction.

How much to tip, how to tip and where to tip

The tip is always
what *you* consider
fair

The how and when
of tipping

Hairdressers tell us that they find it very embarrassing when their clients coyly try to slip the tip into their pocket. The tip is best left in an envelope at the desk with the recipient's name and yours on it. A word of thanks is also appreciated.

Don't forget that if anyone brings you lunch or a beverage, he or she should be tipped too, as should whoever checks your coat and parcels and hands you a robe. These are usually the low men on the totem pole, and they need it more than anyone else.

In the spirit
of Christmas

If you are a steady client at a particular salon, be prepared to give gifts at Christmastime that would make Santa beam. This doesn't necessarily mean breaking the bank. Homemade or baked gifts are always welcome, if you have established a comfortable personal/professional rapport at the salon.

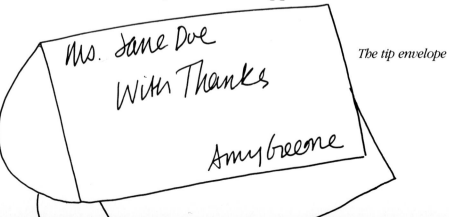

The tip envelope

Ms. Jane Doe
With Thanks

Amy Greene

TIP SHEET: A GUIDE

SERVICE	PRICE	TIP
HAIRCUT	$30–40	$5 up
SHAMPOO	$4–7	$2 up
HAIR WET DOWN	—	$.75
CONDITIONING	$4	Tip included in shampoo tip
SET WITH ROLLERS	$12–16	$2 up
BLOW DRY	$10–16	$2 up
LAMP DRY	$5–7	—
STRAIGHTENING	$60–80	$10 up
PERM	$75–100	$15 up
FIVE WEEK RINSE	$25–35	$5 up
ONE PROCESS COLOR	$60–70	$10 up
TWO PROCESS COLOR	$80–100	$12 up
TOUCH UPS	$35–55	$5 up
FROSTING:		
WHOLE HEAD	$85–95	$12 up
HALF HEAD	$65–75	$10 up
HAIRLINE	$40–50	$7 up

hair hair hair hair

ACKNOWLEDGMENTS

We would like to thank the following hair experts for their generous insights:

Hairdressers

Enrico Vezza, Jr., co-owner of the Astor Place Barber Stylist, 2 Astor Place, New York NY; (212) 475-9854.

Lilian Nepote-Ampala, manager of the Jean Louis David Salon at Henri Bendel, 10 West 57th Street, New York NY; (212) 247-1100.

Angela Campanella, Miss Duval, Victor Friedman, and Eric Jolly of the Kenneth Salon, 19 East 54th Street, New York NY; (212) 752-1800.

Marc de Coster of the Monsieur Marc Salon, 22 East 65th Street, New York NY; (212) 861-0700.

Richard Stein of the Richard Stein Salon, 768 Madison Avenue, New York NY; (212) 879-3663.

Hair colorists

Rosemary Sorrentino
of Julius Caruso,
22 E. 62nd Street,
New York NY;
(212) 759-7574.

Renee Ehni and Albine
of the Kenneth Salon,
19 East 54th Street,
New York NY;
(212) 752-1800.

Robert Renn,
independent colorist,
New York NY.

Edward Moore
of Clive Summers,
654 Fifth Avenue,
New York NY;
(212) 751-7501.

Trichologist (hair/scalp health expert)

Philip Kingsley,
16 East 53rd Street,
New York NY;
(212) 753-9600.

makeup tools

huge powder brush

blusher brush

eye comb/brush

large hairbrush

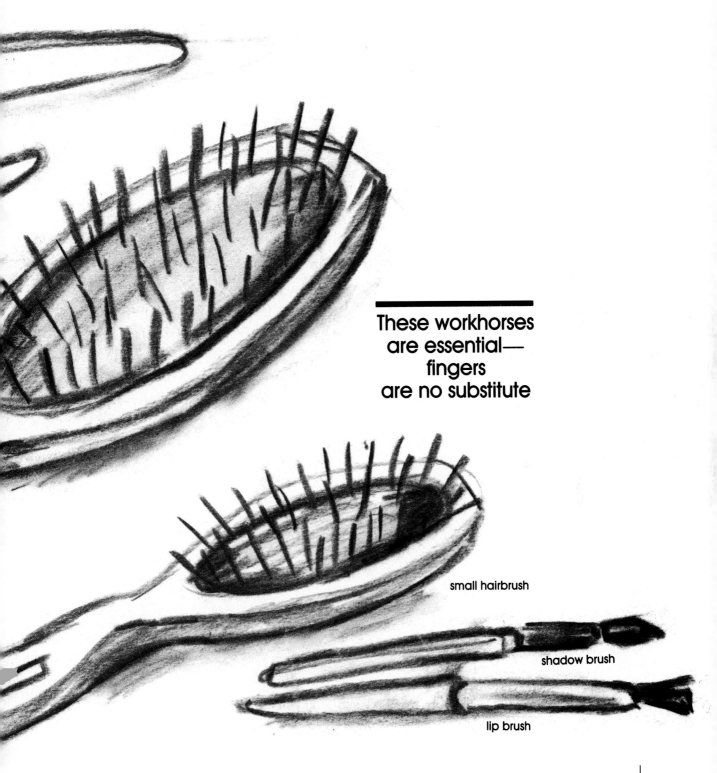

These workhorses
are essential—
fingers
are no substitute

small hairbrush

shadow brush

lip brush

141

ESSENTIAL MAKEUP TOOLS AND COSMETICS

This is not only a comprehensive list of necessary cosmetics, but also a complete makeup tool list. We know through our long experience that the right makeup equipment is just as crucial as the right cosmetics. The simplest tools—a tissue, a cotton swab, the right sized brush—are indispensable to the effect that you want to achieve.

The proper tools and cosmetics in their assigned places save you time and effort. Don't treasure worn out makeup implements as you would the family silver; they don't work as well when they are past their prime, and they are easily and inexpensively replaced.

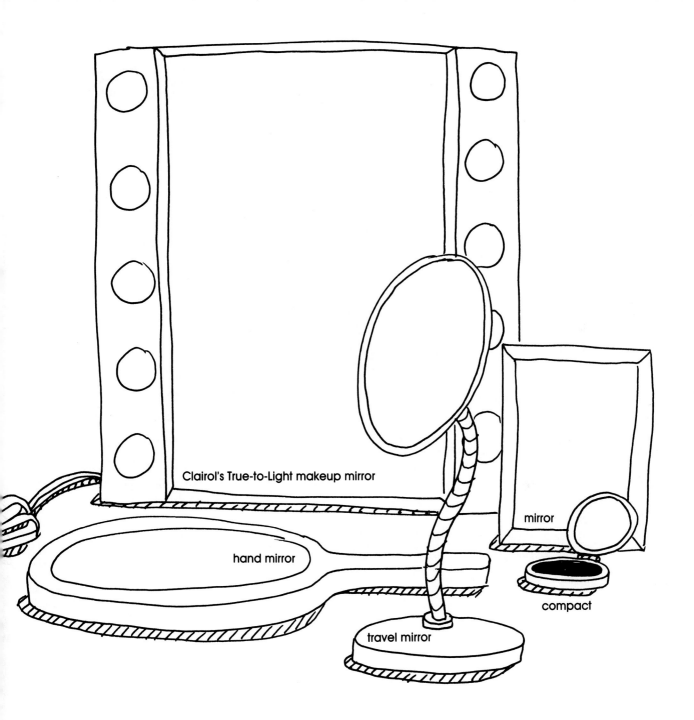

Clairol's True-to-Light makeup mirror

hand mirror

travel mirror

mirror

compact

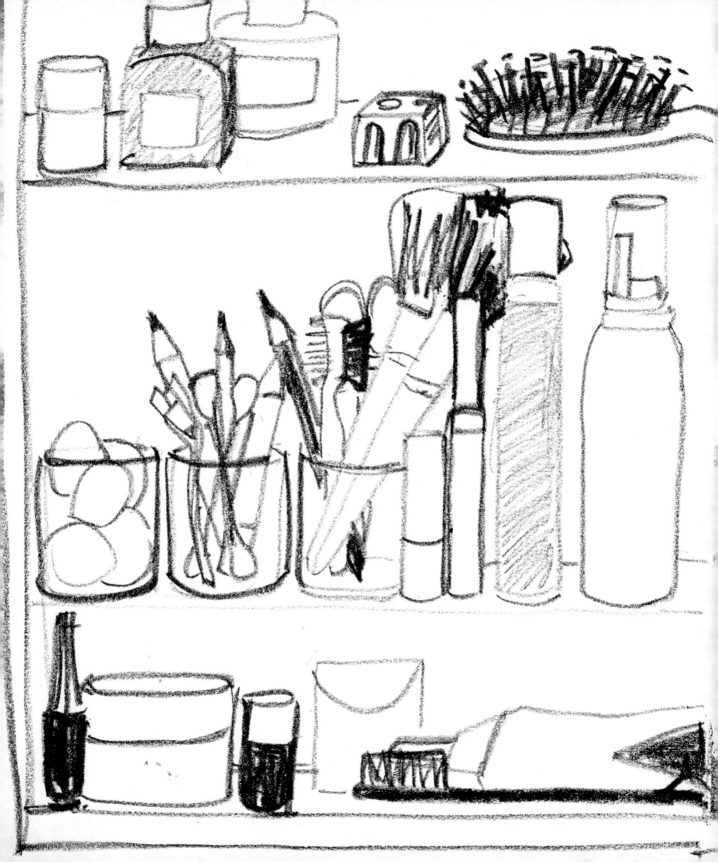

makeup tools

FOR YOUR MEDICINE CHEST OR MAKEUP TABLE

Hair clips, hairband,
ponytail holder or shower
cap to hold back hair
Tissues
Cotton balls—
in covered container
Cotton swabs—
in juice sized glass
Makeup sponge
Brushes—all together
in another glass:
    Shadow brush
    Eyelash/brow brush/comb
    Medium sized blusher brush
    Generous powder brush
    Retractable lip brush
Pencil sharpener for fat and
thin pencils
Eyelash curler
Tweezer
Hairbrush and comb

Cosmetics and toiletries:
    Cleanser
    Toner
    Moisturizer
    Night cream
    Neutralizer
    Foundation
    Concealer
    Rouges: Creamy, liquid,
    powdered
    Powder (loose)
    Eyeshadows
    Eye pencils
    Mascara
    Lipstick, gloss,
    lip balm, lip pencil
    Favorite nail polish
    Nail polish remover
    Nail file, scissors, brush
    Emery board

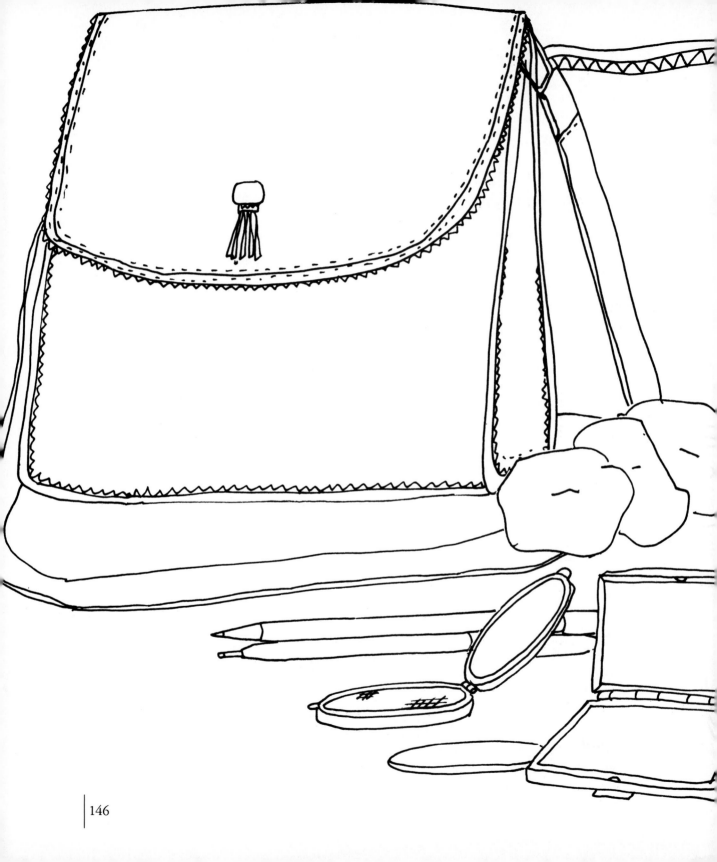

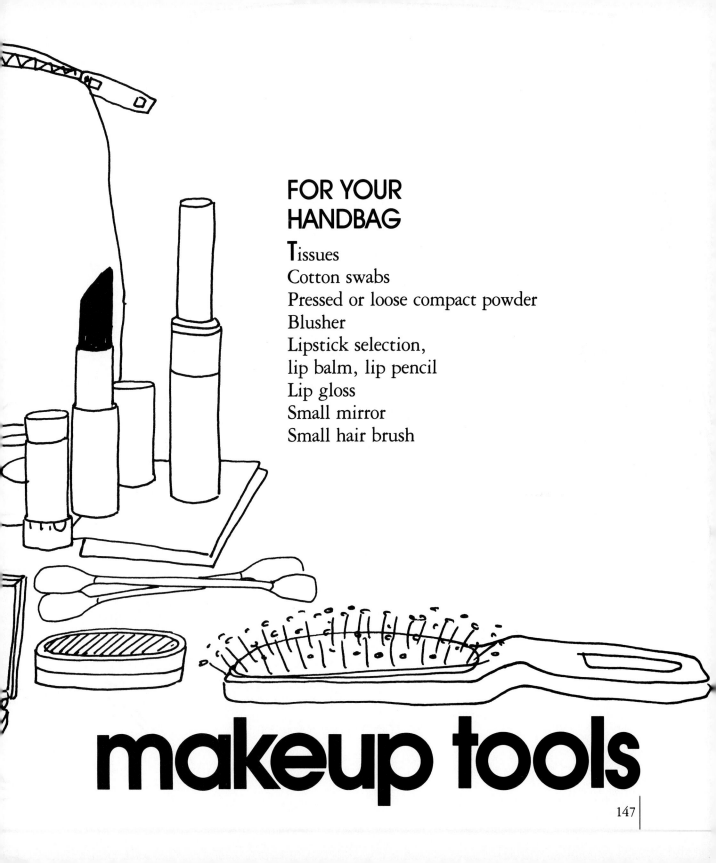

FOR YOUR
HANDBAG

Tissues
Cotton swabs
Pressed or loose compact powder
Blusher
Lipstick selection,
lip balm, lip pencil
Lip gloss
Small mirror
Small hair brush

makeup tools

makeup tools

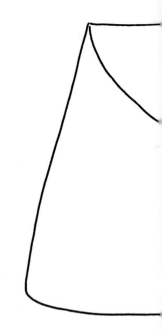

FOR YOUR
EVENING BAG

Same as for everyday bag, plus:
Perfume or fragrance
Blue pencil to line inside rim of eye
Small comb

FOR YOUR
TRAVEL KIT

The same as your everyday medicine chest or makeup table kit. Keep this set up to date so that you are always set to go. Don't borrow individual items from this kit for your everyday use. Otherwise you might forget to replace them and you'll wind up high and dry in the middle of Tibet.

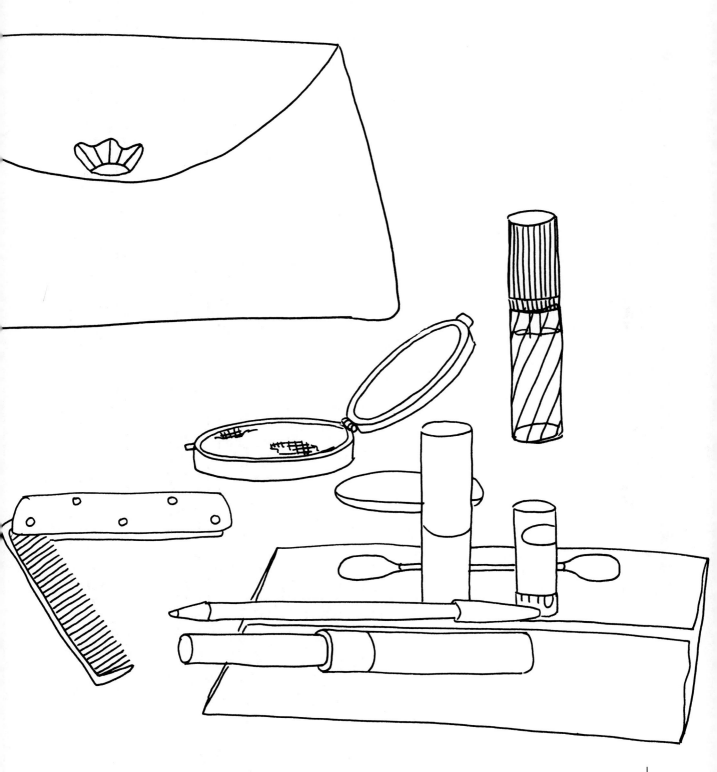

makeup tools

WHEN TO DITCH YOUR MAKEUP

Really edit your cosmetics to keep your supply up to date. Go through them ruthlessly every six months. Eliminate everything you haven't used.

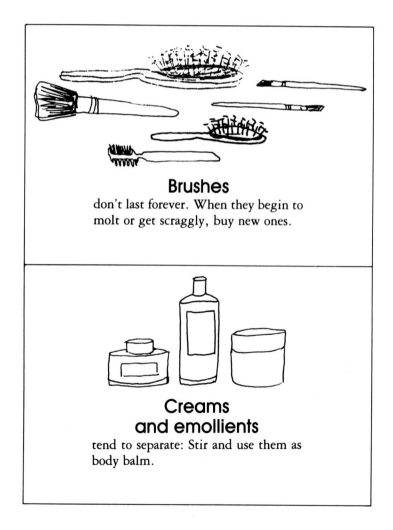

Brushes
don't last forever. When they begin to molt or get scraggly, buy new ones.

Creams and emollients
tend to separate: Stir and use them as body balm.

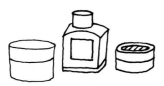

Foundations

also separate: Last year's products should not be used on your face, but on some other part of your body (e.g., leg or ankle to hide veins or discolorations, if you need it).

Fragrances and perfumes

oxidize, turn sour . . . and vanish.

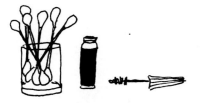

Mascara,

once opened, should be replaced every three months as bacteria accumulate on the brush. Always make sure to screw the top on tightly after using.

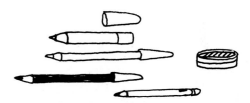

Eyeshadow, eye pencils and rouges

last so long that they become boring. Retire them temporarily. They'll look new again in a few months.

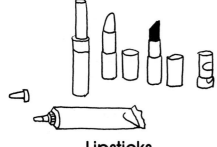

Lipsticks

eventually harden, oxidize, and turn rancid.

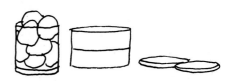

Translucent powder

—loose or pressed—lasts indefinitely. Throw out grimy old *powder puffs* and buy new ones.

the don'ts

AMY GREENE'S UNIMPEACHABLE LISTS OF DON'TS

Read the following lists carefully. Check off the items that are familiar. If you are a perfect person, this chapter is not for you. Otherwise, read on. . .

Face don'ts

Troweled on foundation
Prune dry skin on young women
Rouge in round circles
Unblended streaks of color
Foundation stopping at jaw line
Contouring
Pasty, unmadeup face with overdone eyeshadow and mouth color
Above all, *don't* be rough with your face!

Eye don'ts

Raccoon eyes (concealer improperly blended)
Bloodshot eyes
Overdone shadow
False looking false lashes
Lashes clumped together with mascara
Heavy eyeliner with Cleopatra points
Overpowering sunglasses
Scratched and dirty glasses

Hand don'ts

Uneven, cracked nails
Chipped nail polish
Disco color or dark polish on short nails
Nail polish on little girls
Long, clawlike nails
Silver, green, blue or black nail polish

Hair don'ts

Overteased, overblown hair
Thick blond streaks
Overpermed hair (Bride of Frankenstein look)
Overbleached hair (strawlike)
Punk hairdos—they don't flatter the face
Wiggy looking wigs

Lip and mouth dont's

Neglected teeth
Chapped lips
Lipstick on teeth, glass or mug
Excessive lipstick
Obviously outlined lips

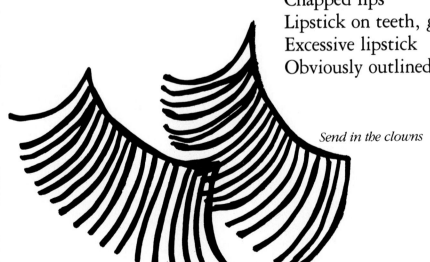

Send in the clowns

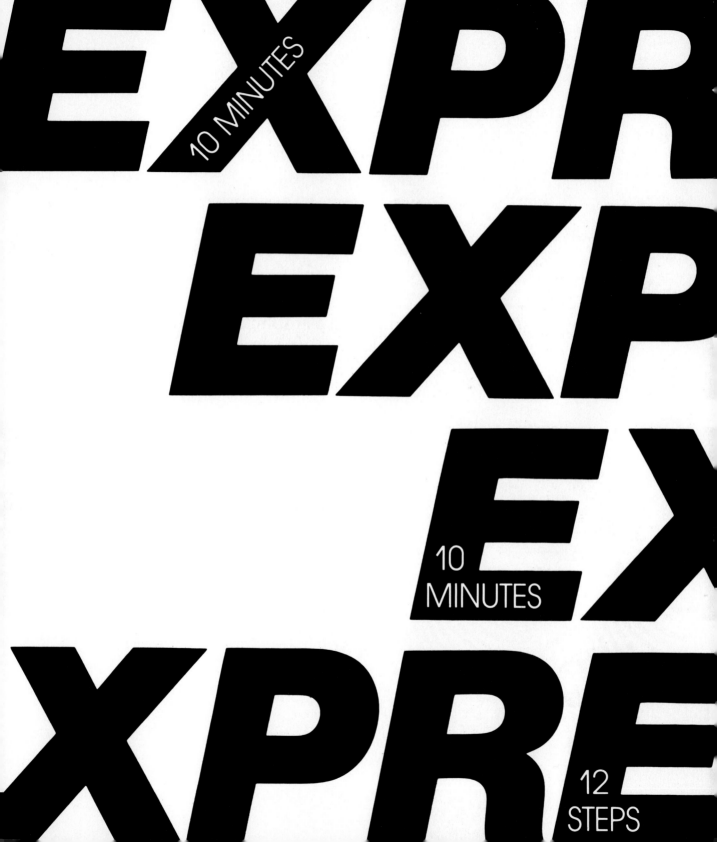

12 STEPS

THE TEN MINUTE, TWELVE STEP MAKEUP

TEN MINUTES TWELVE STEPS

Now that you have absorbed all the Beauty Checkers basic steps and techniques, seriously consider how much time you can comfortably afford to spend on your face every morning.

The most important factors are commitment and concentration. You will see that you can accomplish in ten uninterrupted minutes what it would take you a half hour to do with the phone at your ear.

1 Splash your face with lukewarm water.

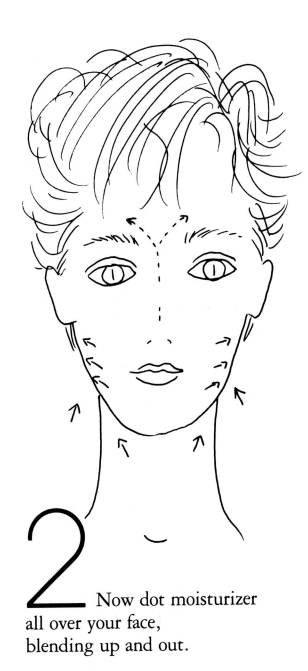

2

Now dot moisturizer
all over your face,
blending up and out.

3

Apply vitamin E stick
or other eye product to the
eye area and laugh lines,
or wherever you are especially dry.

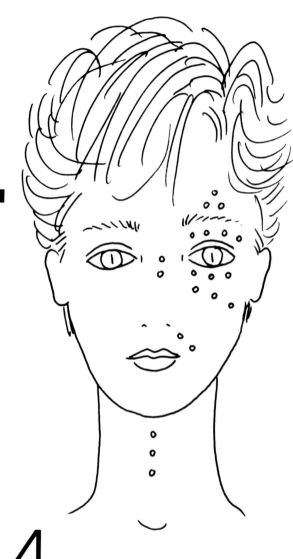

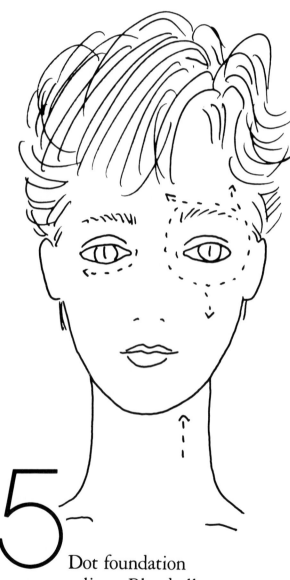

4 Dot neutralizer all over the darkened areas that need correction. Blend.

5 Dot foundation over neutralizer. Blend all over face, not forgetting the eye and the neck area.

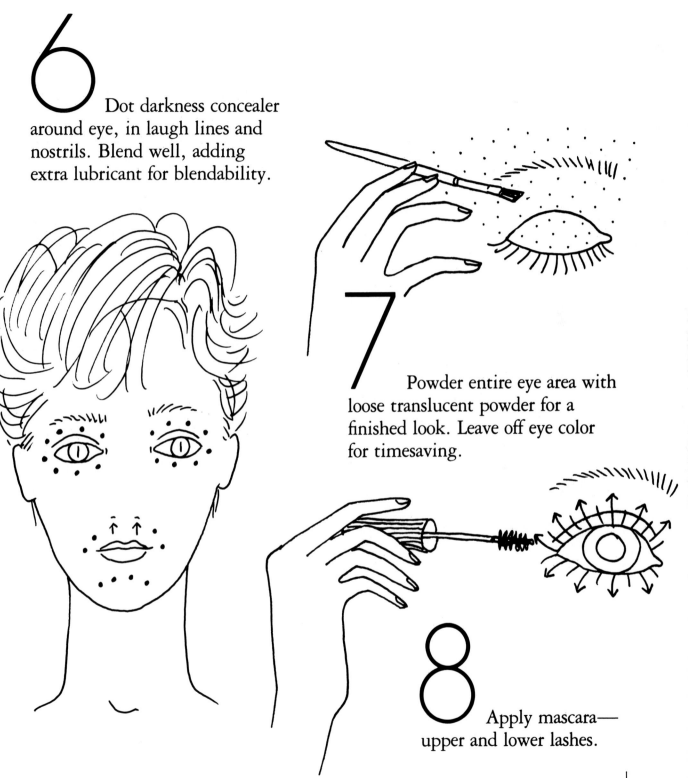

6 Dot darkness concealer around eye, in laugh lines and nostrils. Blend well, adding extra lubricant for blendability.

7 Powder entire eye area with loose translucent powder for a finished look. Leave off eye color for timesaving.

8 Apply mascara— upper and lower lashes.

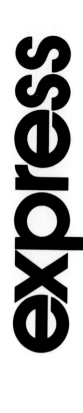

express

9
Use clean cotton ball
to powder over entire face.
Discard cotton ball.

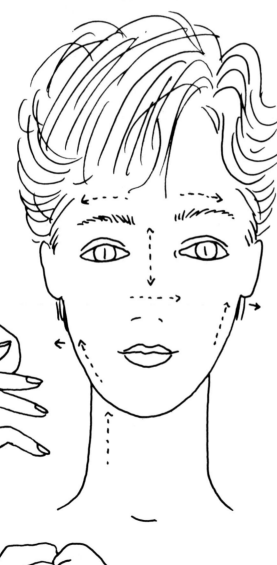

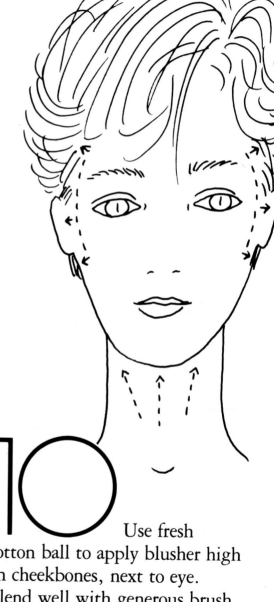

10
Use fresh
cotton ball to apply blusher high
on cheekbones, next to eye.
Blend well with generous brush,
always up and out.

11 Now for the lipstick.
If you outline your mouth, it will last longer.

12 Bend over and brush
hair forward. Straighten up
and brush back. Instant body!

Beauty Checkers

On your day off and on Sundays, practice, practice, practice. Within a week everything in the book becomes rote—and the twenty-minute full makeup becomes *ten minutes*.

your face

notes _____

_____

_____

_____

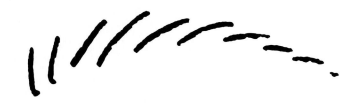

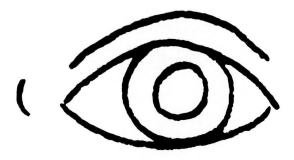

Keep a record of your makeover

Use crayons to color in the face
and eye and use them as a road map

notes _____

_____

_____

_____

glossary

AMY GREENE'S
COSMETICS
GLOSSARY

A

ALCOHOL: Used in many skin products such as soaps, fresheners, astringents. Very drying and should be avoided by all skin types. Even oily skins derive no long term benefit from it.

ALOE VERA: Juice from the aloe plant leaf. Used in gel, cream or lotion form. Soothing to sunburned skin.

ANTISEPTICS: Substances which inhibit the growth of bacteria on the skin, such as alcohol, hexachlorophene, peroxide and witch hazel (extremely drying).

ASTRINGENTS: Products intended to make the pores of the skin seem smaller. They contain aluminum salt, a chemical which causes a slight swelling, temporarily "swallowing" the pores and creating this *illusory* effect.

B

BABY OIL: See mineral oil.

BALSAM: A substance used in some shampoos, conditioners and cream rinses. Coats the hair shaft with a clear layer, adding body to the hair and helping it retain moisture. Smells wonderful!

BASE: See foundation.

BEESWAX: A form of wax often used in cosmetics.

BIRTHMARKS: Moles present at birth; strawberry marks (which usually fade) and port wine stains (which do not); both are hemangiomas, or blood vessel accumulations. Some success has been achieved in fading birthmarks by laser.

BLEACHING: The process by which the color is removed from the hair.

BLEMISHES: A word widely used to refer to unsightly spots or imperfections of the skin.

BLENDING: The technique of gently smoothing cosmetic products onto the skin in small feathery strokes. Should always be done in an upward and outward direction.

BLUSHER, PRESSED POWDER: Colored powder, pressed in a case, to be applied over a bed of translucent face powder. Has good lasting properties.

BOTTLED WATER: Derived from natural springs all over the world, containing minerals that may be beneficial in cleansing the system when consumed regularly. Recommended for use on hair and face as a final rinse when the local water is too hard or polluted.

BROKEN CAPILLARIES: Dilated blood vessels, caused by pregnancy, birth control pills, liver diseases, sun exposure, extremes of temperature and hereditary tendency.

C

CALAMINE: A soothing solution of minerals used in foundations, concealer and cosmetic creams with an opaque finish. Also used in lotion form to soothe irritated skin.

CAMPHOR: A vegetable product easily absorbed by the skin which has antiseptic qualities and is used in some cosmetics and lip balms. Produces a mild tingling sensation.

CASTILE SOAP: A good, inexpensive soap made mostly of olive oil.

CERTIFIED COLOR: A dye used in edible products as well as in cosmetics. The government guarantees its safety when used in certain limited quantities. The FDA reviews the list periodically.

CLAY: A mineral found in powders, face masks and makeup bases. It is harmless and benefits oily skin.

CLEANSERS: Creams, liquids or lotions used to remove grime and makeup from the face that can be rinsed or tissued off.

COCOA BUTTER: Coconut oil, in solid form, used in

many face creams, sun creams and lotions. Softens the skin.

COCONUT OIL: An oil often used in soaps; it helps produce a good lather. Double the rinse cycle as all oil leaves a film.

COLD CREAM: The great-grandmother of all modern creams, cold cream is an excellent cleanser. The name came from the cool feeling left on the skin when the water in the cream evaporated.

COLD SORES: Viral ulcerations that may appear on the lips, the nose, the chin or in the mouth. They occur when the body's resistance is lowered.

COLLAGEN: The naturally produced substance that gives everyone's skin its elasticity. It is weakened and altered by aging and the sun. Used in minuscule quantities as an ingredient in some creams and lotions, and injected by some dermatologists to plump up lines on the face.

COLORING: The generic word for "hair dyeing."

COMB/BRUSH: A two sided beauty utensil with one side toothbrushlike, the other a tiny comb. Either side is used to separate, fluff out or smooth brows and lashes.

CONTOURING/SHADING: An ineffective method of using light and dark rouges in an effort to accentuate and "create" facial bone structure. Never works.

CORNSTARCH: Absorbs water and is soothing to the skin. Used in some depilatories and powders and as a thickener in some cosmetics.

COSMETICS PUFFS/ COTTON BALLS: Sterilized cotton or synthetic equivalent in measured rolls, useful for anything to do with makeup application, removal or blending.

COTTON SWABS: Small plastic or cardboard sticks tipped at each end with a tiny pad of tightly wound cotton. Invaluable for blending and removing eye makeup and for correcting cosmetics mistakes of all kinds.

COWLICK: An obstinate clump of hair that grows in its own direction and cannot be persuaded to yield.

CRISCO: Pure vegetable shortening in a can that is excellent for use as a night cream and for protection against harsh weather. Recommended by dermatologists and plastic surgeons. Totally nonirritating.

D

DARKNESS CONCEALER: A creamy lotion or paste intended to lighten dark areas of the face. Best applied over foundation in tiny dots, and well blended.

DEODORANT SOAP: This contains antibacterial chemicals, good for the body but useless for the face where there are no odor producing glands. These chemicals can cause skin discoloration if the soap is used prior to sunning.

DEPILATORIES: Chemicals that dissolve the hair at skin level. The more effective ones have an odor and can irritate. They have been known to cause skin burns, rashes and even headaches.

DETERGENT (in soaps or shampoos): Degreases the skin and hair; thorough rinsing is imperative.

DYE: See also "certified color." Substance derived from mineral, vegetable or animal sources that is used in cosmetics to give the desired color.

E

EMULSIFIERS: Chemical agents which enable the process of emulsion to take place and are added to cosmetics for this purpose.

EMULSION: The state that occurs when two or more normally nonmixable liquids are so thoroughly shaken together that they appear homogenized.

ENDPAPERS: Tiny squares of paper used with rollers for setting the hair. They act as a cushion between hair and rollers, to prevent indentation.

ESTROGEN: A hormone from the ovaries. Often used in night creams for the "mature" skin. Consult with your doctor before using as it can be absorbed into the system.

EYEBROW PENCIL: A soft pencil with a thin point used to fill in and define eyebrows. Heavily used, it creates an artificial and aging look. A #2 writing pencil is an excellent (and economical) substitute.

EYELINER, LIQUID: Applied with its own tiny brush. Used at the very edge of the lid close to the lash. Never inside the eye.

EYELINER, PENCIL: Thin pencil used to line inside rims of eye (upper and lower) or to outline. Must be nonirritating.

EYE MAKEUP REMOVER: Products to remove all eye makeup, including mascara. Available in liquids, creams, gels and oil soaked pads.

EYESHADOW, CREAM: Not as long lasting as powdered shadow, but for those with crepey eyelids or contact lenses, they are an effective alternative. Available in many shades.

EYESHADOW, PENCILS: In a fat version useful as eyeliner or shadow. In thin version, to be used as eyeliner inside or outside the eye. There are also retractable pencils in various sizes; the thinner they are, the easier to use.

EYESHADOW, POWDERED: Easiest to work with. Pans of pressed colored powder, in any shape, size or hue, frosted or matte. To be applied (in combinations of two or more) with a small brush, over a powdered eyelid, and blended. Disintegrates easily. Not portable. Available in all price ranges.

F

FACE GELS: Instant face color, containing alcohol, dries superfast, staining whatever it touches. To be used in conjunction with moisturizer.

FACE MASKS: Products which are said to cleanse the skin, minimize wrinkles or tighten pores when rinsed or peeled off. The temporary feeling of tightness and coolness that they give creates this illusion.

FACIAL HAIR: This hair can be removed by waxing, plucking or depilatories, but will grow back rapidly. Electrolysis is more effective and longer lasting but costly. We believe that the shaving of facial hair for women should *never* be done.

FALSE LASHES: Human or synthetic hair attached to a soft, pliable transparent strip of plastic; it is glued to the edge of the lid close to the natural lash.

FOUNDATION: (Also called "base.") A viscous product in varying shades of skin color to be applied over moisturizer in small quantities and blended. Helps even out color and texture. Comes in oil or water base, cream, emulsion, gel, liquid, cake or stick.

FRECKLES: Excesses of pigment producing cells which tend to darken and multiply in the sun. Often genetic, they are usually associated with fair complexions and redheads.

FRESHENERS/TONERS: Lotions designed to remove the greasy residue of cleanser from the skin. Not as drying as astringents because they are not as strong.

G

GLYCERIN: Substance used in a number of cosmetics and other toiletries to make them spread better. Terrific in hand lotions. May dry some skin, however.

H

HAIR: A protein called *keratin,* which is also what composes your nails and the top layer of your skin.

HAIR COLOR RINSE: Chemical product that changes

the color of the hair by coating only the shaft, not the roots. Lasts only until it oxidizes, grows out or is rinsed out.

HAIR CONDITIONER: Product designed to restore shine and manageability to the hair. Crucial to chemically processed, very thick or tangle prone hair.

HAIR STRAIGHTENING: Chemical process which eliminates whatever natural curl, frizz, wave or kink you may have in your hair. Should only be done by a professional.

HAND CREAMS: Moisturizers for the hands. Usually heavier and more fragranced than facial lubricants.

HARD WATER: Water which is found in most urban parts of the country, containing calcium and other mineral salts. Requires triple rinsing time to get rid of soapy residue.

HARD WATER SOAPS: Soaps containing extra alkaline properties useful in keeping the skin clean where the water is too hard to lather with regular soaps.

HENNA: Vegetable dye widely used as a red tint for the hair. It is messy; repeated use causes color buildup. Suits some hair perfectly, while dulling others. Does not cover gray.

HIGHLIGHTER: An iridescent cosmetic cream, pencil, liquid or powder to be used on the eyelid or to dramatize facial bone structure in evening makeup. Looks artificial in daylight.

HIGHLIGHTING: The process of lightening groups of hair strands to contrast with the actual hair color.

HYDROGEN PEROXIDE: Chemical substance often used in hair dyes. Lightens the hair and helps the color applied to develop. Can dry the skin.

HYPOALLERGENIC: A term used to describe products containing no known irritants. Imprecise, however, as nothing is truly "hypoallergenic."

I

IRIDESCENCE: The shimmery finish to some lipsticks, powders, foundations, rouges, blushers, nail polish and eyeshadow that is derived from a mineral called "mica." Most effective in evening makeup. Can cause allergic reaction.

IRRITANTS: Chemical ingredients in cosmetic products and toiletries that may cause allergic reactions.

K

KERATIN: A protein from which the top layer of the skin is formed; also the hair and nails.

L

LANOLIN: One of the oils most consistently used in cosmetics. Helps prevent evaporation of water. Sometimes causes allergic reactions.

LASH CURLER: A curved metal, rubber or Teflon tipped implement with scissor type handles. Used prior to mascara application to curl the top lashes. The original design is perfection.

"LAUGH LINES": Lines running from the nose to the outer corners of the lips. They are often inherited and can appear at a very young age. Application of a darkness concealer on top of foundation will minimize them.

LEMON: Often used in either natural or artificial form in cosmetics. Natural lemon has good degreasing qualities for hair in final rinse. Also an excellent stain remover.

LIGHT: Essential to checking makeup, be it fluorescent, incandescent, or, best of all, natural daylight.

LIP BRUSH: A small brush used to outline the lips with lipstick and to spread the color evenly.

LIP GLOSS: Color either in

little jars or in transparent tubes with sponge tip applicator. To be used over lipstick or alone; imparts shine and sometimes color. Lasts briefly on the lips.

LIP PENCIL: A soft pencil in reddish shades used to outline and define the lips before applying color.

LIP PRIMER: Also known as lip balm. A lubricating stick containing less wax than lipstick, to be applied to the bare lips as a moisturizer and as a base for lip color.

LIPSTICK: Color in a tube, made primarily of oil and wax with a red staining certified dye; flavoring and perfume are sometimes added. Available in regular, frosted, medicated and sheer forms in a huge choice of colors. Lasts longer than gloss.

LIQUID ROUGE: Tinted liquid to be used directly over foundation or moisturizer. Should be blended immediately to prevent staining.

LIVER SPOTS: Flat brown spots, usually found on sun-exposed areas of mature skin. They are an accumulation of pigment producing cells, and actually have nothing whatever to do with the liver.

LUBRICATING STICK: Concentrated moisture in lipstick form to be used in very dry areas such as around the eyes and on laugh lines.

Used nightly as an eye cream, it is less likely to cause puffiness than regular moisturizers. Fine for lubricating specific dry areas on oily skins.

M

MASCARA: Product used to darken the lashes and make them appear longer and fuller. Must be thoroughly removed at night (see eye makeup remover). Comes in plastic tube or glass bottle with spiral brush; in cake form to be dampened with its own tiny brush; and in a squeeze tube also with its own brush. The latter is usually waterproof.

MASK OF PREGNANCY: A brownish discoloration sometimes found on the cheeks, temples and noses of women who have an excessive amount of estrogen in their systems. Sun makes it worse. Fades slowly but not completely.

MILK: Often used, in addition to other ingredients, in face masks, bath products and other toiletries. Has soothing properties. Must be rinsed very thoroughly.

MINERAL OIL: The most commonly used oil in cosmetics. Has no smell and is nonirritating.

MOISTURIZER: Cream or lotion containing mineral oil, water and other lubricating substances that the pores can

absorb. Applied to a slightly damp skin, helps keep the body's moisture from evaporating too fast. Also acts as a barrier against pollutants.

MOUSSE: A foam that comes out of an aerosol can, this is the 1980s answer to setting lotion. Used on wet hair to help sculpt it. Since it traps pollutants, daily shampoos for mousse users are imperative.

N

"NATURAL": In cosmetic terms, this means absolutely nothing; to preserve the shelf life of any product, it must contain some amount of preservative.

NEUTRALIZERS: (Also known as underbases or primers.) Viscous aqua or lavender products to apply after moisturizer and before foundation, to tone down complexions that are too ruddy or too sallow. Should not be used on their own.

NIGHT CREAM: Lubricant to apply to the face after washing it at night. Heavier than daytime moisturizer, it tends to take longer to be absorbed. May cause puffiness in the eye area.

NONALKALINE: Soaps suited for dry or delicate skin.

O

OLIVE OIL: A vegetable oil used in the manufacture of

castile and "olive oil" soaps. Though harmless in soap, should not be used as a suntan oil because it will not block the burning rays and you'll cook.

OIL BASED FOUNDATION: Contains a larger percentage of oil than water for better coverage; perfect for dry skin.

OXIDATION: The natural process by which all color fades or changes through contact with the air and light.

P

PABA: Para aminobenzoic acid. The acid found in the vitamin B complex that is used in many sunscreens to prevent damage from the sun, and as a mild local anesthetic. May cause allergic reactions.

PENCIL SHARPENERS: Available everywhere in small, medium and large sizes. Essential that the aperture correspond to the size of the pencil. A blunt sharpener will ruin your pencil.

PERMANENT WAVING: A chemical process which makes straight hair wavy, gives limp hair body, and makes thin hair thicker. Best done by an experienced professional or at home by following the directions on the package *exactly.*

PETROLEUM JELLY: A harmless but heavy protective covering that sits on the surface of the skin.

PLACENTA EXTRACT: From animals; it is used in some creams and lotions allegedly to revitalize the "mature" skin.

PLUCKING: Pulling out of individual hairs, usually of eyebrows. Must be done with a very accurate tweezer in a bright light or hair will snap at the surface of the skin. Very temporary in its effect, but useful because it can be done on a daily basis.

POWDER, LOOSE/PRESSED: See translucent powder.

PROGESTIN: A derivative of the female hormone progesterone which is used in some creams and lotions for the "mature" skin. Check with your doctor before buying, because it can be absorbed into the system and is expensive.

R

ROLLERS: Cylindrical objects used with setting lotion on clean wet hair to give the hair body, height, wave or curls. They come in every imaginable size, the gentlest being mesh or foam covered. Rollers should always be used with endpapers. Electric rollers can be used on dry hair.

ROUGE, CREAM: Tinted cream intended to be used directly over foundation or moisturizer. Apply several times for desired color.

S

SCALP CONDITIONER: Product to remedy scalp problems; it should be recommended by a skilled hair professional. If the problem persists, a dermatologist should be consulted.

SCRUBBING GRAINS: Abrasive agents composed of either wheat germ, oatmeal or powdered almonds in a cream or paste base. Used to remove surface impurities from the skin, and to scrub off dead cells. To be used infrequently, with caution, and never around the eyes or on dry or sensitive skin.

SESAME OIL: Used in suntan lotion; it blocks out 30 percent of the harmful sun rays.

SHAMPOOS: Hair cleansers that are available in great variety for every hair type. The less detergent they contain, the better. Read the label.

SHAVING: Cuts off the hair at skin level, causing it to grow back quickly and stubbly. For women, suitable for use only on legs and underarms.

SILICONES: Minerals used in lotions, face creams and shampoos to help prevent moisture from evaporating too fast from skin and hair. Silicone is also used by certain dermatologists and plastic surgeons to plump up wrinkles and improve body contours.

STREAKING: More dramatic than highlighting, this is a bolder way of lightening hair strands. It involves considerable upkeep and is best done by a professional.

SUNSCREENS: Lotions or gels that screen out more of the sun's burning rays than regular suntan products. They do not provide total protection and must frequently be reapplied. Many contain PABA, to which some people are allergic. The SPF or sun protection factor, on a scale of up to 20, is on the package. Always read before buying.

SUPERFATTED SOAPS: Their high fat content makes them especially effective for cleansing dry skin. Examples are Basis, Oilatum and Dove.

T

TONER: See freshener.

TRANSLUCENT POWDER, LOOSE: Unpressed powder in a box or a jar. It is an ideal finish, hiding flaws and extending the life of a makeup. Will not clog the pores or change color.

TRANSLUCENT POWDER, PRESSED: Same face powder pressed into a compact. Ideal for touch ups during the day; spillproof when carried in your cosmetics kit.

TRANSPARENT SOAPS: Their glycerin and alcohol content tends to dry the skin if not rinsed thoroughly.

TWEEZERS: A small metal implement used to pull out individual hairs. Tweezers come in a number of styles, with differently shaped tips. Throw them out when they no longer grip.

T ZONE: The facial area with the highest concentration of oil glands. Anchor shaped, it runs down the center of the face from forehead to chin and across the chin.

W

WARTS: Virally induced, benign growths which spontaneously disappear after a period of two years or so. Can be removed by a doctor.

WATER BASED FOUNDATION: Contains a larger percentage of water than oil (but some oil, however delicate, is the essential blending agent in *all* foundations). Provides less coverage than oil based foundation, it feels lighter on the skin.

WAX: The emulsifying agent that unites all substances used in most cosmetics and toiletries, such as creams, lotions, lipsticks, nail polish and eye products.

WAXING: An efficient way of temporarily removing facial and body hair. Warm wax is spread over the necessary area, and quickly stripped off when it cools, pulling the hairs out with it.

WITCH HAZEL: The only natural, botanical astringent approved by the F.D.A., its distinctive odor comes from Hamamelitannin, which is the active ingredient.

Z

ZINC OXIDE: Totally opaque mineral with soothing properties that is insoluble in water. Sometimes used in cosmetics, it is a totally effective sunscreen—a lifeguard's best friend.